U0295370

年龄与医疗费用

从谜题到证据

Aging and
Medical Expenses:

from Mystery to Evidence

主 编 金春林 李 芬

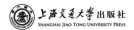

上海交通大学出版社
SHANGHAI JIAO TONG UNIVERSITY PRESS

内容提要

本书结合上海市老年人口医疗服务利用的特点，采集老年人口医疗费用的相关数据，分析临终前不同阶段医疗费用的特点，模拟终身医疗费用，探索医疗费用随年龄增长的变化规律，为合理配置医疗资源、科学厘定医疗保险费率、控制不合理的费用增长、提高资源的利用效率提供循证依据，提出医疗服务供给侧改革以及应对老龄化的医疗费用筹集、分配和使用策略。

图书在版编目(CIP)数据

年龄与医疗费用：从谜题到证据/金春林，李芬主编. 一上海：上海交通大学出版社，2018
ISBN 978-7-313-19150-2

Ⅰ.①年… Ⅱ.①金… ②李… Ⅲ.①老年人-医疗费用-研究-上海 Ⅳ.①R197.1

中国版本图书馆 CIP 数据核字(2018)第 049692 号

年龄与医疗费用：从谜题到证据

主　　编：金春林　李　芬		
出版发行：上海交通大学出版社	地　　址：上海市番禺路 951 号	
邮政编码：200030	电　　话：021 - 64071208	
出 版 人：谈　毅		
印　　制：上海盛通时代印刷有限公司	经　　销：全国新华书店	
开　　本：710 mm×1000 mm　1/16	印　　张：16.5	
字　　数：275 千字		
版　　次：2018 年 7 月第 1 版	印　　次：2018 年 7 月第 1 次印刷	
书　　号：ISBN 978-7-313-19150-2/R		
定　　价：85.00 元		

上海市领军人才项目（项目编号：059）

上海市第四轮公共卫生三年行动计划重点学科建设项目循证公共卫生与卫生经济学
（项目编号：15GWZK0901）

英国外交部中国繁荣基金项目"人口老龄化对上海医疗费用的影响
（中英合作研究）"（项目编号：16SS23）

本书由上海市卫生和健康发展研究中心主持出版

编　委　会

序

上海是座繁华而又充满活力的大都市,街道两旁摩天大楼林立,东南西北各式车流交汇,全国各地的英才集聚。作为全国经济、金融、贸易以及航运中心,加上近期提出的发展科技创新中心的目标,上海的建设和发展欣欣向荣。然而,物质和商业文明高度发达的同时,上海"老"得也是遥遥领先。2015 年,上海市 2 400 万常住人口中,60 岁以上老年人占比为 19.5%,户籍老年人口占比已超过 30%。

上海是我国期望寿命最高的城市,老龄化呈现出高龄化、慢病化、失能化、空巢化、少子化五个特点。高龄化、慢病化和失能化意味着医疗需求增加,而空巢化、少子化则意味着家庭养老功能下降。与老龄化相伴而来的是健康状况的下降和医疗服务需求的上升。人民群众日益增长变化的健康需求与以急性期治疗为主要功能的传统医疗卫生服务体系间的不平衡、不充分不断凸显。如何应对老龄化的挑战,亟需循证依据来支持决策。不同年龄阶段的病种结构、医疗服务利用和医疗费用、资源消耗结构有什么差异?医疗卫生资源配置应如何以需求为导向进行相应调整?上海市居民临终前医疗行为和医疗费用有什么特征?是否出现临终前医疗费用突增现象?增加多少?哪些费用出现增长?这些变化是否合理?有无过度与不足?老龄化不断加剧的背景下,医疗卫生资源和费用需求量是多少?解开这些谜底,寻找循证依据,正是开展本项研究的初心。

本书首先呈现现有老年人口医疗卫生体系基本框架,在此基础上分析我国及上海市老年人口医疗服务体系和保障现状及主要经验、存在的问题和面临的挑战。基于上海市卫生服务调查、上海市卫生和计划生育委员会信息中心健康信息网平台数据，详述了老年人口医疗需要、服务利用、医疗费用的现状及特点，探索了临终前医疗服务利用和医疗费用规律，分析医疗费用的影响因素，总结了国际上不同卫生体系代表性国家如德国、英国和日本等国应对老龄化的卫生体系实践经验及启示，最后提出了完善卫生筹资及合理控费政策、优化医疗资源配置和利用结构、探索老年医疗服务模式的政策建议。本书也将主要研究结果翻译成英文，附于书后。

　　研究的开展获得了政府各部门及相关单位的数据与智力支持，深表感谢。项目组成员精诚合作，厚厚的讨论稿、加班后昏黄的路灯、半夜手机上亮起的绿色信号，与书中的文字一起存储在心里。"健康上海2030"提出健康期望寿命达到全球城市先进水平，"健康老龄化"势在必行；近日，国务院批复上海市城市总体规划，打造宜居、宜业的社区服务圈，医疗、养老等服务必不可少。

　　谨以此书献给所有关心老年健康服务的相关人士，以及我们每个人终将遇见的老年。

上海市卫生和健康发展研究中心主任

2017 年 12 月 24 日

目　录

第一章

前　言

【导读】

　　我国老龄化速度逐渐加快、程度不断加深，如何在有限的资源条件下满足老年人口的医疗需求，已成为迫在眉睫的问题。为应对这个挑战，我国开展了医疗服务体系的系列改革，但进行符合老年人口医疗服务需求和利用特点的体系设计还需要更系统、全面的循证决策依据。本章梳理了国内外年龄与医疗费用关系的研究，发现老年人医疗费用的确高于60岁以下群体，但费用结构发生变化，护理费用增长明显。老年人发生死亡的比例高，学术界所称的"接近死亡效应"（即临终前发生的医疗费用高）对老年群体的总体医疗费用影响大。虽说是普遍规律，但年龄与卫生保健服务的利用和支出间的关系是多变的。在一些高收入国家，人均卫生保健的支出约在75岁以后明显下降。"接近死亡效应"在不同国家差别较大，卫生系统的影响在临终阶段表现得尤为明显。然而，上述研究证据多来自发达国家，与我国的文化准则、卫生体系差异大，因此，基于本土数据开展研究显得尤为必要。

中国已于 20 世纪末进入老龄化社会,人口结构老化已成为社会发展的巨大挑战,而如何保障老年人口健康是其中的突出问题。开展年龄与医疗费用影响研究显得极为重要、必要和迫切。国家统计局发布的第六次全国人口普查主要数据显示,2010 年,我国 60 岁及以上人口占比 13.26%(17 765 万人),其中 65 岁及以上人口占比 8.87%(11 883 万人)。同 2000 年第五次人口普查相比,60 岁及以上、65 岁及以上人口的比重分别上升 2.93 和 1.91 个百分点[①]。而根据《2015 年国民经济和社会发展统计公报》,2015 年,我国老龄化程度进一步加深,60 岁及以上人口占比 16.1%(2.22 亿人),65 岁及以上人口占比 10.5%(1.44 亿人)[②]。老年人群医疗需求大,且随着人口老龄化程度不断加深,需求将进一步释放,医保基金压力增加。而我国现阶段人均医疗资源紧张,医疗体系负担较重,若不解决现有筹资模式的结构性问题,医保基金将难以为继,将给政府和社会带来前所未有的压力。因而,满足老年人群需求并控制其医疗费用,必须统筹考虑。目前各地逐渐开始探索构建医养结合下的多层次的老年护理保障制度体系,而制度的设计必须以老年人口医疗需求的结构为导向,以符合老年人群医疗服务利用的规律为基石。在这样一个背景下,开展老年人群医疗服务需求与医疗服务利用分析,探究医疗费用随年龄变化的规律,以期为完善卫生筹资模式、调整卫生资源结构提供数据支撑,就显得尤为重要。

一、国内外年龄与医疗费用关系研究主要结果

随着年龄增长和健康状况的变化,相应医疗需求也会发生改变,老年人口个体间的身体状况差异导致医疗需求多样化[③]。从社会的角度看,老龄化是一个持续的进程,伴随着社会经济发展、收入提高、医疗技术进步、

---

① 中华人民共和国国家统计局.中国统计年鉴 2015[M].中国统计出版社,2015.
② 中华人民共和国国家统计局.中华人民共和国 2015 年国民经济和社会发展统计公报[N].人民日报,2016-03-01(010).
③ Brooks-Wilson A R. Genetics of healthy aging and longevity[J]. Human Genetics,2013,132(12):1323—1338.

医疗保障体系改革等变化,老龄化对医疗费用的影响是在各项因素的共同作用下发生的。众多学者对老龄化等相关因素对医疗费用的影响进行了分析,但由于假设理论、内涵界定和选用方法的不同,研究结论不尽一致。

(一) 老年人医疗费用增长、结构改变

多项现状研究表明,老年人口人均医疗费用及其增长速度高于其他年龄组,护理费用增长迅速。Waldo 和 Lazenby(1984)[1]、Buchner、Wasem 等(2006)[2]发现,人口老龄化将加重医疗费用负担,原因是随着年龄增加,健康状况下降,医疗服务需求和费用增加。Reinhardt 等(2003)[3]认为,年龄增长导致的健康水平下降推高了医疗费用,65 岁及以上人群的医疗花费是 34～44 岁组的 3 倍多。Lassman 等(2014)[4]研究发现,老年人口的人均医疗费用是儿童的 5 倍。也有研究认为,老年人口的医疗费用主要是护理费用。Temkin-Greener(1992)等[5]认为,若排除护理费用,医疗费用随着死亡年龄的增长而减少。Hartman 等(2008)[6]对 1987—2004 年美国卫生总费用的研究发现,老年人人均卫生费用远高于儿童和中青年人群,但老年人与中青年人群人均卫生费用之比却从 1987 年的 6.9 倍下降到 2004 年的 5.7 倍;研究认为,造成比例下降的原因是居家护理(nursing home care)费用的同期上涨幅度远低于人均卫生费用幅度,而居家护理费用占 85 岁及以上人口卫生费用的绝大部分。

国内关于老年人口医疗费用的相关研究多数集中在人口老龄化与医疗费

---

① Waldo D R, Lazenby H C.Demographic characteristics and health care use and expenditures by the aged in the United States：1977—1984[J].Health Care Financing Review, 1984，6(1)：1—29.

② Buchner F, Wasem J."Steeping" health expenditure profiles[J]. Geneva Papers on Risk & Insurance Issues & Practice, 2006，31(4)：581—589.

③ Reinhardt U E.Does the aging of the population really drive the demand for health care？[J].Health Aff (Millwood), 2003,22(6)：27—39.

④ Lassman D, Hartman M, Washington B, et al.US health spending trends by age and gender：Selected years 2002—10[J].Health Aff (Millwood), 2014,33(5)：815—822.

⑤ Alemayehu B, Warner K E.The lifetime distribution of health care costs[J]. Health Serv Res,2004, 39(3)：627—642.

⑥ Hartman M, Catlin A, Lassman D, et al.U.S.health spending by age, selected years through 2004[J].Health Affairs, 2008，27(1).

用增长的关系方面。一些研究认为,老年人口对医疗服务需求较高,因而,随着老龄化程度加深,医疗费用将快速增加。医疗费用增长受多重因素影响,年龄结构变化有影响但没有其他因素大。王超群(2014)认为,老龄化会缓慢地提高老年人口潜在的医疗服务需求,而收入提高、医疗保险扩张和医疗技术进步等因素则会快速释放老年人口的卫生费用[①]。马爱霞等(2015)研究发现,性别、年龄、婚姻状况和城乡身份等因素均对老年人的医疗卫生支出具有显著影响[②]。余央央(2011)利用 2002—2008 年 20 个省份的面板数据研究发现,老龄化仅解释了人均医疗支出增长变化中的 3.9% 和人均医疗支出增长率变化中的 5.7%[③]。封进等(2015)利用中国营养与健康调查 1991—2011 年的数据考察城乡居民医疗支出的年龄效应,发现城市居民人均医疗支出随年龄显著增加,而农村居民的人均医疗支出随年龄增长的趋势并不明显,1990—2010 年由人口老龄化和城乡差距缩小带来的医疗费用年均增速为 2.7%,贡献了期间总费用增长率 13.3% 中的 1/5[④]。

横截面数据分析存在的缺陷是混合了不同的出生队列,不同年龄阶段的人均医疗费用差异可能与其暴露因素有关;而队列研究所得出的差异混杂了医疗服务价格、医疗技术进步等其他因素的影响。Alemayehu 和 Warner (2004)[⑤]采用现时寿命表和横截面医疗费用数据模拟美国密歇根蓝盾保险参保人员的终身医疗费用,得出各个年龄组的期望医疗费用,获得了不同生命阶段医疗费用的变化趋势。结果显示,平均约 1/3 的医疗费用发生在 40～64 岁;65 岁及以上的老年人,医疗费用占终身医疗费用的 1/2;对于 85 岁及以上的老年人,期望医疗费用占终身医疗费用的 1/3 以上。

(二) 医疗费用具有接近死亡效应

医疗费用具有"接近死亡效应"(Proximity to Death),临终前医疗费用高

---

① 王超群. 老龄化是卫生费用增长的决定性因素吗? [J]. 人口与经济,2014(3): 23—30.

② 马爱霞,许扬扬. 我国老年人医疗卫生支出影响因素研究[J]. 中国卫生政策研究,2015,8(7): 68—73.

③ 余央央. 老龄化对中国医疗费用的影响——城乡差异的视角[J]. 世界经济文汇,2011(5): 64—78.

④ 封进,余央央,楼平易.医疗需求与中国医疗费用增长——基于城乡老年医疗支出差异的视角[J].中国社会科学,2015(3): 85—103.

⑤ Alemayehu B, Warner K E.The lifetime distribution of health care costs[J]. Health Serv Res.2004,39(3): 627—642.

于生存者的医疗费用。Blakely 等(2014)[①]对新西兰 2007—2009 年医疗费用数据(包括住院、门诊、药品、检验)进行分析，按照性别和年龄分组，统计死亡前 6 个月、12 个月的医疗费用。结果显示，存活居民 6 个月的人均医疗费用在 498 美元(10~14 岁组)至 6 900 美元(90~94 岁组)不等；临终前 6 个月的医疗费用要高出 10 倍，婴儿组和高龄老人(80 岁及以上)人均大于 3 万美元。据世界卫生组织综述，不同国家的"接近死亡效应"相差很大，例如澳大利亚和荷兰用于临终者最后一年的卫生支出，约占全部卫生保健费用的 10%，而美国约为 22%。

梳理针对接近死亡效应的研究结果，发现接近死亡效应受距离死亡时间、年龄、疾病、费用结构和地域的影响。

(1) 距离死亡时间。距离死亡时间越近，发生医疗费用的概率越大、费用越高(Seshamani 和 Gray，2004)[②]。

(2) 年龄。McGrail(2000)等对 1987—1988 年、1994—1995 年加拿大 65 岁以上人群的临终 6 个月的急性治疗费用、长期护理费用研究发现，年龄越大，医疗费用的死者生者之比越小：65 岁组为 16.6，75~76 岁组为 8.4，90~93 岁组下降为 2.5[③]；Polder 等(2006)[④]、Shugarman 等(2008)[⑤]分别对荷兰、美国的医疗费用进行分析，认为较年轻的死亡者平均医疗费用高于年纪较大的死亡者。

(3) 费用结构。Shugarman 等(2008)[⑥]对加拿大的研究发现，高年龄组临

① Blakely T, Atkinson J, Kvizhinadze G, et al. Health system costs by sex, age and proximity to death, and implications for estimation of future expenditure [J]. New Zealand Medical Journal，2014,127(1393)：12—25.

② Seshamani M, Gray A. Ageing and health-care expenditure：The red herring argument revisited[J]. Health Economics，2004，13(4)：303.

③ McGrail K, Green B, Barer M L, et al. Age, costs of acute and long-term care and proximity to death：evidence for 1987—88 and 1994—95 in British Columbia.[J]. Age & Ageing，2000，29(3)：249—253.

④ Polder J J, Barendregt J J, Van O H. Health care costs in the last year of life-the Dutch experience[J]. Social Science & Medicine，2006，63(7)：1720—1731.

⑤ Shugarman L R, Campbell D E, Bird C E, et al. Differences in Medicare expenditures during the last 3 years of life.[J]. Journal of General Internal Medicine，2004，19(2)：127—135.

⑥ Shugarman L R, Bird C E, Schuster C R, et al. Age and gender differences in medicare expenditures and service utilization at the end of life for lung cancer decedents. [J]. Womens Health Issues，2008，18(3)：199.

终前更多地利用护理和舒缓疗护,门诊和住院费用相对较少。不同费用之间具有替代作用,舒缓疗护的增加显著降低了转院和 ICU 的发生,相应的舒缓疗护费用增加,住院费用及其他类型医疗费用降低[①]。

(4) 疾病种类。Wong 等(2011 年)[②]对疾病别临终医疗费用分析发现,癌症花费最高,心肌梗死花费最低。

(5) 地域影响。不同国家的"接近死亡效应"相差很大。由于临终费用受年龄别、疾病别、费用结构的影响,不同情境下的老龄化社会,接近死亡效应也会呈现不同的结果。

(三) 其他外生因素与医疗费用关系研究

人口社会学特征(婚姻状况、家庭人口数、教育程度、职业类别、收入等)、个人健康特征和行为、医疗保险类型等也可能对医疗费用产生影响。Felder 等(2001)[③]研究发现,收入、医疗保险等对临终前医疗费用产生影响,享受补充保险的人群较普通保险覆盖人群产生更高的临终前医疗费用,低收入家庭在生命两年末期的医疗服务花费较高收入家庭低。Hartman 等(2008)[④]认为,美国医疗费用的增长更多归因于参保人群的增加,而非年龄结构的变化。Dormonta 等(2006)[⑤]测算显示,医疗费用增长仅 3.4% 归因于年龄变化,医疗技术进步带来的医疗行为的改变是老龄化对医疗费用影响的 3.8 倍。Poldera 等(2006)[⑥]认为,死因变化、疾病的严重程度较年龄更有助于预测医疗费用。Poldera 等通过对 210 万人(荷兰人口的 13%)的调查研究发现,人口老龄化对卫生总费用的影响小于科技进步带来的影响,而人口骤增对医疗卫生系统可持续发展带

---

① Hashimoto H, Ikegami N, Shibuya K, et al. Cost containment and quality of care in Japan: is there a trade-off? [J]. Lancet, 2011, 378(9797): 1174—1182.

② Wong A, van Baal P H, Boshuizen H C, et al. Exploring the influence of proximity to death on disease-specific hospital expenditures: A carpaccio of red herrings [J]. Health Economics, 2011, 20(4): 379—400.

③ Felder S, Meier M, Schmitt H. Health care expenditure in the last months of life [J]. Journal of Health Economics, 2000, 19(5): 679—695.

④ Hartman M, Catlin A, Lassman D, et al. U.S. Health spending by age, selected years through 2004[J]. Health Affairs, 2008, 27(1): w1—w12.

⑤ Dormonta B, Grignon M, Huber H. Health expenditure growth: Reassessing the threat of ageing[J]. Health Econ. Health Economics, 2006, 15(9): 947—963.

⑥ Polder J J, Barendregt J J, van Oers H. Health care costs in the last year of life — The Dutch experience[J]. Social Science & Medicine, 2006, 63(7): 1720—1731.

来的影响不可小觑，卫生体系结构对医疗费用也产生较大影响。美国预计，婴儿潮人群的老龄化会导致护理院费用的增加（Hartman 等，2008）[①]，但实际增长低于预期，可能是居家护理和社区护理的发展所产生的替代作用。

二、学术界的争议及原因

（一）年龄与医疗费用关系的主要争议点

国外关于老龄化与医疗费用关系研究主要集中在三个方面。

一是老年人口与其他年龄组平均医疗费用的比较研究，包括横断面研究和队列研究。从平均医疗费用来看，老年人口的平均医疗费用普遍高于其他年龄组。时间序列数据比较发现，老年人口平均医疗费用增长速度也相对较快。但如果排除护理费用，医疗费用随死亡年龄的增加而减少。美国出现医疗费用增长低于预期，是因为居家护理和社区护理的发展对医疗服务的替代作用，降低了老年人口的总体医疗费用水平。从中也可以推断，服务体系结构是医疗费用的重要影响因素，将影响老龄化实际产生的作用。

二是分析年龄与距离死亡时间两个因素对医疗费用的作用程度。少数研究结果认为，接近死亡效应的存在使得老龄化对医疗费用的"净影响"小，甚至为负相关。世界卫生组织 2015 年发布的《关于老龄化与健康的全球报告》指出，卫生保健费用最高的阶段往往是在生命最后的 1～2 年，但不同的国家之间差别较大。

三是分析年龄与其他影响因素变化的情况下，老龄化对医疗费用的影响。对医疗费用影响较大的因素包括收入提高、参保人数增加、医疗技术进步等，除少数研究认为老龄化对医疗费用的影响为负或不相关，普遍研究认为年龄结构变化对医疗费用的归因贡献度不一，但普遍低于技术进步等因素。我国多项研究认为，老龄化对医疗费用的影响是显著的，但归因贡献度差异较大，从3.9%至20%不等。

（二）研究结论产生差异的主要原因

学术界的观点形似迥异，然而界定研究概念和厘清实证研究后仍有规律

---

① Hartman M, Catlin A, Lassman D, et al. U.S. health spending by age, selected years through 2004[J]. Health Affairs, 2008, 27(1): w1—w12.

可循。首先,研究结论取决于医疗费用口径是否包含长期护理费用。当医疗费用中包含长期护理费用时,年龄对医疗费用增长影响更大。其次,当研究对象纳入的影响因素不同时,结论自然有差异。以 Zweifel 等为代表的学者关注的是当期望寿命增加时对医疗费用的内生影响,即固定其他影响医疗费用的因素,仅研究年龄因素对医疗费用的影响;而以 Buchner 和 Wasem 等学者为代表的研究,除年龄之外还考了其他因素的影响。再次,在不同国家和地区,老龄化对医疗费用的影响本身存在差异。老龄化与医疗费用的关系受文化风俗、医疗服务体系、卫生筹资体系等因素的影响,不同国家、地区的研究结论存在地域差异。卫生系统的影响,如卫生体系、激励机制、针对脆弱老年群体的干预措施以及文化准则方面的差异,对医疗费用的影响大;该差异在临终阶段表现得尤为明显。因而,建立整合性的医疗服务、增加长期照护,有利于提高老年人口健康程度,降低医疗费用。

三、本书拟回答的问题

截至 2014 年末,中国老年人口(60 岁及以上)约 2.12 亿人(占总人口数的15.5%),预计到 2025 年,老年人口占比将达到 20%,这意味着我国应对老龄化的时间相对其他国家更少,这对政策制定的反应性提出了严峻的要求。从文献综述来看,在不同时期和不同国家,老龄化对医疗费用的影响程度不一,老龄化与医疗服务利用和医疗费用的关系并非单一的,而是受卫生系统本身的影响,因而,开展老龄化与医疗费用关系研究,根据当地卫生系统、文化背景等特点来制定相关政策非常必要。目前国际上关于老龄化对医疗费用影响的证据主要来自发达国家,我国基于大样本的研究很少,在老龄化给医疗服务体系带来的挑战方面,缺乏本土研究证据。上海是我国最早进入老龄化的地区之一,在信息化建设方面处于全国前列,开展全样本研究的基础较好。在服务体系方面,上海市将老年人口服务机构作为资源配置时的重点考虑问题;在具体措施上,大力发展老年医疗护理服务。2015 年,社区卫生服务机构、老年护理院和二级综合性医院等共有老年护理床位 2.3 万张。此外,上海市人力资源与社会保障局已于 2017 年起开始试行长期护理保险制度。

本书基于大数据,全面了解上海市常住人口医疗服务利用和医疗费用的数量和构成,重点分析临终就诊机构和医疗费用的特点,将老年人口医疗服务利用和医疗费用的特点应用于上海市卫生资源配置规划,从而更好地满足老年人口医疗服务需求，提高资源的利用效率。本书将医疗费用数据与生命表模型相结合，模拟终身医疗费用，探索医疗费用随年龄增长的变化规律，预测老龄化程度加深给医疗费用带来的变化，为完善卫生筹资制度、建立老年护理保障制度提供数据支撑。

第二章

老年医疗服务体系和保障现状概览

【导读】

　　2015 年,上海市 60 岁及以上户籍人口比例为 30.2%,65 岁及以上人口占比为 19.6%;全国层面上,60 岁及以上的老年人口占比达 10.3%,可见上海老龄化程度高、发展速度快,这对政策制定的反应性提出了严峻的要求。上海市政府非常关注老龄化问题,上海市卫生和计划生育委员会在制定区域卫生规划时重点规划为老服务体系,并着手制定老年护理规划;上海市人力资源和社会保障局拟制定老年护理保障制度。本章对上海市老年人口的医疗服务提供及医疗保障政策进行了系统梳理,基于对卫生、民政、人保、财政等部门的关键知情人及多位专家、学者的访谈,总结了当前服务体系的特点、存在的问题及下一步的发展方向。结果显示,老年人口医疗服务需求具有水平高、以慢性病为主、康复护理及临终关怀需求显著的特点。目前,上海市为老年人口提供医疗服务的方式主要有三种:根据需求评估分级提供差别化服务、整合性的医疗卫生服务以及在社区搭建平台推进医养结合。上海市医疗保障体系包括托底层、基本层、补充层和自愿层四层,每个层次中都有倾斜性设计。相对其他年龄群体来说,老年群体的医疗保障体系设计具有医保筹资负担较小、医疗费用报销程度较高、有一定的医疗负担风险防范机制等特点。当然,上海市老年医疗服务体系和保障体系还存在着管理体制条块分割、资源配置不甚合理、医疗保障制度设计不够完善、浪费与不合理服务利用并存等问题。

一、老年人口医疗服务需求特点

（一）医疗服务需求水平高于全人群

老年人口生理机能衰退，健康水平下降，各种慢性疾病发生率较高，导致老年人口对医疗服务的需求较一般人群高。随着人口老龄化程度加剧，诸如癌症、脑卒中、老年痴呆症等慢性疾病所累及人口的绝对数字将持续增加[1]，老年人口的医疗服务需求会进一步释放。2010 年中国慢性病监测数据显示，74.20% 的 60 岁及以上老年居民自报或检测出至少患有 1 种常见慢性病[2]。2013 年国家卫生服务调查数据显示，我国 60 岁及以上老人两周患病率是全人群的 2.36 倍，慢性病年患病率是全人群的 2.16 倍。从上海地区来看，60 岁及以上老人两周患病率是全人群的 2.40 倍，慢性病年患病率是全人群的 1.84 倍；老年人口两周就诊率、年住院率分别为 44.49%、12.14%，远高于全人群的平均水平（21.91%、6.69%）。由数据可见，老年人口的医疗服务需求明显高于全人群平均水平。

（二）疾病特点以慢性病为主，病程长

以慢性病为主、病程长是老年人口的主要患病特点。2012 年中国居民死因监测报告显示，65 岁及以上老年人群慢性病死亡人数已占到总死亡人数的92.6%，慢性病是老年人的主要死因。随着年龄增长，老年人口的慢性病患病率增加，生活不能自理的比例也在升高[3]。上海市卫生和健康发展研究中心副主任黄玉捷指出，不同年龄段老年人的自理能力差别较大，服务需求也就不同，老年人口的医疗服务需求呈现分段式特征：60～70 岁，以医疗服务需求为主，主要是到门诊拿药；70～80 岁，护理需求比例升高，医疗服务需求主要为治

---

① Prince M J，Wu F，Guo Y，et al. The burden of disease in older people and implications for health policy and practice. Lancet[J].2015,385(9967)：549—562.

② 崔娟,毛凡,王志会.中国老年居民多种慢性病共存状况分析[J].中国公共卫生，2016(1)：66—69.

③ 周国伟.中国老年人自评自理能力：差异与发展[J].南方人口,2008(1)：51—58.

疗服务;80岁以上老年人主要为护理需求,医疗服务需求相对较少。

不同的疾病种类和所需要的医疗服务类型密切相关,不同类别疾病对医疗服务需求的影响差异较大①。复旦大学人口与发展政策研究中心主任彭希哲认为,可以将慢性病细分为三类,对应不同的服务需求:一是常见慢性病,主要是利用门诊慢性病处方服务;二是癌症等大病,以住院治疗服务需求为主,也有部分护理需求;三是脑卒中、老年痴呆等失能、伤残类大病,主要是康复、护理需求。

(三) 康复、护理、临终关怀需求剧增

随着年龄的增长,不但老年人口的健康水平有所下降,其失能率和残障率也会迅速增加。2010年,全国高龄老年人(75岁及以上)中失能者为928万人,低龄老年人(60岁及以上且在75岁以下)中失能者为1 146万人;高龄老年人(75岁及以上)中残障者为289万人,低龄老年人(60岁及以上且在75岁以下)中残障者为217万人②。第二次全国残疾人抽样调查数据显示,60岁及以上老年人中,残疾人数为4 416万人③,占老年人口的24.43%。这些失能、残障、残疾老人生活自理能力不足,需要专门的长期照护服务,对护理及康复服务需求较大。

临终期患者以老人居多,且随着人口老龄化,终末期慢性病老人、高龄老人临终者数量会逐渐增多。临终期患者的生命质量普遍不高,承受身体及精神的双重煎熬,存在着各种心理问题和不良情绪,单纯治疗服务意义不大,不仅会加重家庭的负担,也造成医疗资源的浪费。临终关怀服务作为预防、治疗服务之外的一种针对临终患者的补充服务,在老年群体中的潜在需求较大。

二、上海市老年人口医疗服务体系现状

(一) 医疗服务机构总体架构

上海市整个医疗服务提供机构主要有医院、基层医疗卫生机构、公共卫生

---

① 王翌秋,王舒娟.居民医疗服务需求及其影响因素微观实证分析的研究进展[J].中国卫生政策研究,2010(8):55—62.

② 饶克勤,钱军程,陈红敬,等.我国人口老龄化对卫生系统的挑战及其应对策略[J].中华健康管理学杂志,2012,6(1):6—8.

③ 中国残疾人联合会.2006年第二次全国残疾人抽样调查主要数据公报(第二号).[EB\OL].2007-11-21. http://www.cdpf.org.cn/sjzx/cjrgk/200711/t20071121_387540_3.s.html.

机构和其他机构,其中既有公立机构,又有非公立机构(见图2-1)。面对老年人的预防、医疗、护理和康复需求等,不同类型机构提供具有一定针对性的医疗卫生服务,各类机构的分工不同,如表2-1所示。

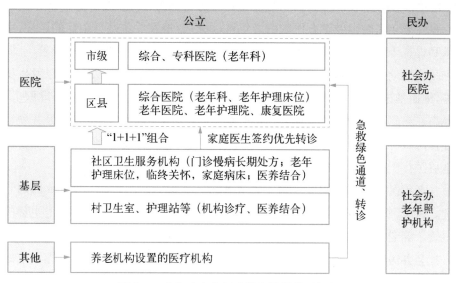

图 2-1 上海市老年医疗服务提供体系框架

表 2-1 服务内容与服务提供机构对应表

服务类别 \ 机构类别	设置老年科的医院	老年医院/老年护理院	基层医疗卫生机构	家庭病床	养老机构	社区托养机构
预 防	＊	＊＊	＊＊＊	＊	＊＊	＊＊
医 疗	＊＊＊	＊＊	＊＊	＊	＊	＊
护 理	＊	＊＊＊	＊＊	＊＊	＊＊	＊
康 复	＊	＊＊＊	＊	＊	＊	＊
临终关怀	—	＊＊	＊＊	—	＊	—

注：① 这里的养老机构专指设置医疗机构的养老机构,一般设置老年护理床位;社区托养机构以日间照料中心、长者照护之家、综合为老服务中心等为代表,一般与社区卫生服务中心签约,为老人提供医疗卫生服务。

② ＊表示该类服务由该类机构提供的程度。其中,"＊＊＊"代表该类服务主要由该类机构提供,"＊＊"代表该类服务部分由该类机构提供,"＊"代表该类服务仅有少部分由该类机构提供。

针对老年人的一般诊疗、护理、康复需求,主要由基层医疗卫生服务机构和养老机构设置的医疗机构提供,包括在门诊开具的慢病长期处方、常规检查,居家护理设立家庭病床和养老院病床,由基层医疗卫生机构提供培训和指导服务。而针对老年人的住院护理及专业性康复需求,主要由老年护理院、康复机构、设置老年护理床位的医疗机构来提供。随着年龄增长,老年人的健康风险增加,医疗需求更为突出,与之相对应的老年医疗提供主体是二级以上的专科性老年医院以及综合医院的老年科,承担老年人危重疑难杂症的诊疗、手术和检查等服务。针对较大比例老年人在生命终末期的临终关怀需求,上海市政府推动建立舒缓疗护(临终关怀)项目,试点机构主要为基层医疗卫生机构,继而推进设立机构和居家舒缓疗护床位,主要提供姑息治疗和护理服务,提高临终患者生命质量。此外,针对老年人的基本和重大公共卫生服务项目等预防服务被证明具有成本效益,如老年人健康体检、大肠癌筛查等,主要由基层医疗卫生服务机构提供,接受公共卫生机构的指导。

老年医疗服务提供机构由于其服务内容不同,分别由不同的行政部门管理。医院、基层医疗卫生机构、公共卫生机构和老年护理院等主要由卫生部门主管。养老机构和日托中心等社区居家服务机构则由民政部门负责管理。另有社会办医院和老年照护机构等,主要在行业层面,分别受卫生部门和民政部门管理。

在医疗服务体系方面,2015 年,上海市共有医疗卫生机构 5 016 个,其中医院 338 个,占全部机构数的 6.74%;其中护理院 23 个,占全部机构数的 0.50%;共有社区卫生服务机构 1 035 个,占比 20.63%;门诊部占比 12.62%;妇幼保健机构和专科疾病防治机构占比均为 0.42%。其他机构数为 2 968 个,占比为 59.17%,占比最高。2015 年,上海市全部医疗机构中共有 12.28 万张床位,其中大多数分布在医院,占比为 84.30%(其中护理院占总床位数的 5.4%),分布在社区卫生服务机构的占 13.9%,其他机构占比都不超过 2%。如表 2-2 所示。

表 2-2　2015 年上海市医疗卫生机构数量和床位情况

机 构 类 别	机 构 数		床 位 数	
	个	占比(%)	张	占比(%)
医院	338	6.74	103 526	84.30
其中: 护理院	25	0.50	6 645	5.41
社区卫生服务机构	1 035	20.63	17 099	13.92

续　表

机构类别	机　构　数		床　位　数	
	个	占比(%)	张	占比(%)
门诊部	633	12.62	—	
妇幼保健机构	21	0.42	1 317	1.07
专科疾病防治机构	21	0.42	148	0.12
其他	2 968	59.17	723	0.59
合计	5 016	100.00	122 813	100.00

注:"其他"主要包括专业公共卫生机构和疗养院、卫生监督检验所(站)等相关卫生机构。

2015 年,上海市共有卫生技术人员 17.02 万人,医院中的卫生技术人员占比达到了 68.87%(其中护理院占比 1.08%),社区卫生服务机构占比 16.74%,门诊部占比 4.88%,妇幼保健机构和专科疾病防治机构占比分别为 1.58%和 0.65%。卫生技术人员中,执业(助理)医师 6.31 万人,注册护士 7.54 万人,其中,医院执业(助理)医师和注册护士分别为 3.86 万、5.79 万人,占 61.09%和 76.77%(其中护理院占总人数的比例分别为 0.58%和 0.79%),社区卫生服务机构分别占比 19.05%和 13.75%,门诊部分别占比 6.43%和 4.32%,妇幼保健机构分别占比 1.65%和 1.70%,专科疾病防治机构占比最少,不到 1.00%。如表 2-3 所示。

表 2-3　2015 年上海市卫生人力资源数量及构成

机构类别	卫生技术人员		其　　中			
	人数	占比(%)	执业(助理)医师(人)	占比(%)	注册护士(人)	占比(%)
医院	117 209	68.87	38 559	61.09	57 911	76.77
其中:护理院	1 835	1.08	368	0.58	593	0.79
社区卫生服务机构	28 498	16.74	12 021	19.05	10 376	13.75
门诊部	8 310	4.88	4 056	6.43	3 262	4.32
妇幼保健机构	2 695	1.58	1 039	1.65	1 280	1.70
专科疾病防治机构	1 107	0.65	564	0.89	374	0.50
其他	12 370	7.27	6 879	10.90	2 235	2.96
合计	170 189	100.00	63 118	100.00	75 438	100.00

按照服务地点划分,老年人的医疗卫生服务分为机构服务、社区服务和居家服务。机构方面,截至 2016 年 6 月,上海市共有老年护理机构 331 家(包括以服务老人为主的社区卫生服务机构),老年护理床位 2.62 万张。其中公办社区卫生服务中心 242 家(73.11%),共有护理床位 13 031 张(49.73%);公立护理院 12 家(3.63%),共有护理床位 2 820 张(10.76%);社会办(私立)护理院 34 家(10.27%),共有护理床位 7 689 张(29.35%);设置护理床位的二级综合性医院 43 家(12.99%),共有护理床位 2 661 张(10.16%)。近年来,上海市分批逐步推进部分二级公立医院转型发展,目前已成立 3 家康复医院。社区居家医疗护理服务方面,截至 2015 年底,上海市共新建 5.27 万张家庭病床,设置 19 家社会办护理站开展居家护理服务。此外,上海市在 2012 年和 2014 年作为市政府实事项目推进舒缓疗护(临终关怀)工作,截至 2014 年底,全市在以社区卫生服务中心为主的 76 家医疗机构中共开设居家和机构舒缓疗护床位 1 700 余张(其中机构床位 890 张),为各类临终患者提供居家和机构相结合的舒缓疗护(临终关怀)服务。截至 2016 年 6 月,上海市老年护理机构和老年护理床位的具体分布情况如表 2-4 所示。

表 2-4　上海市老年护理机构和老年护理床位分布(2016 年 6 月)

机 构 类 别	老年护理机构		老年护理床位	
	数量	占比(%)	数量	占比(%)
二级医院	43	12.99	2 661	10.16
社区卫生服务中心	242	73.11	13 031	49.73
公立护理院	12	3.63	2 820	10.76
社会办护理院	34	10.27	7 689	29.35
合计	331	100.00	26 201	100.00

注:二级医院指设置老年护理床位的二级医院。

(二) 医疗服务提供方式及探索

目前,上海市针对老年人并无统一的医疗服务提供方式,根据服务内容的不同,主要结合政策文件对各类服务标准的要求开展服务。医疗服务主要由老年人根据需求自主选择各级各类医院或基层医疗卫生机构就诊;机构护理服务主要在老年护理院和老年照护机构中,由专业护理人员提供较为专业化的服务;家庭病床等居家护理主要由医疗机构的医务人员上门提供专业医疗护理服务。值得注意的是,三级医院设有针对部分老年人服务的特需病房(干部保健等),可能影响整个老年人群体的就医公平性。

虽然在全市层面并未广泛实施统一的医疗服务提供方式,但各区县均针对老年医疗服务开展相应探索,具体来说有以下几种模式。

一是根据需求评估分级提供差别化服务。开展老年照护统一需求评估有助于明确服务内容,确定补偿比例,保障老年人的服务可及性和可负担性。徐汇区是上海最早开始试点老年照护统一需求评估体系的区县之一,根据60岁以上老人的失能程度、疾病状况、照护情况等进行评估,确定一至六级照护等级(见表2-5),作为老人享受相应的社区居家老年照护、养老机构和老年护理机构服务的前提和依据。截至2015年12月底,徐汇区老年照护统一需求评估试点工作已提出申请1 664人次,其中居家养老595人、高龄老人居家医疗护理365人、机构养老556人、护理院148人,完成评估904人[①]。

表2-5 老年照护需求评估等级及对应服务内容

照护等级	服 务 内 容
照护一级	生活照护30小时/月
照护二级	生活照护40小时/月＋护理服务1小时/周(孤老)
照护三级	生活照护40小时/月＋护理服务2小时/周
照护四级	养老机构服务:如选择社区居家养老服务,生活照护50小时/月＋护理服务2小时/周
照护五级	养老机构服务:如选择社区居家养老服务,生活照护50小时/月＋护理服务5小时/周
照护六级	养老机构内设护理床位或老年护理机构服务:如选择社区居家养老服务,同五级内容

二是整合性的医疗卫生服务。部分老年护理医院在提供护理服务的同时,针对老年疾病和需求特点优先发展心血管科、神经内科、康复科,与三级医院相关科室合作开展老年病的治疗及康复研究。如东海老年护理医院[②]作为

---

① 徐汇区试点老人照护统一需求评估 在哪养老看报告[EB/OL]. http://www.sh.xinhuanet.com/2016-01/28/c_135051998.htm.

② 舒鉴明.养老医疗护理康复"四位一体"服务再扩容[N].东方城乡报,2015-04-14,A06.

集老年医疗、老年护理、老年康复、临终关怀为一体的综合性医院,其养老、医疗、护理、康复"四位一体"的老年护理服务模式得到各方肯定。

三是在社区搭建平台推进医养结合。《关于加强社区综合为老服务中心建设的指导意见》(沪老龄办发〔2016〕5号)中提出,鼓励社区综合为老服务中心与周边医院、社区卫生服务中心、康复护理等机构合作,引入社区卫生服务站(点、室)、护理站或其他康复机构的服务,或与已有的医疗服务机构综合设置,加强在社区层面的医养结合。提供基本医疗护理服务、康复护理专业指导、健康监测和指导、用药提醒和指导、陪同就诊、取药等服务。虹口曲阳社区打造"一站式"综合为老服务平台①,集合了传统的窗口咨询、文化娱乐等服务,同时引入了养老服务综合评估、社区家庭医生制、家庭养老介入服务等新功能。该中心的社区卫生服务点是曲阳社区卫生服务中心设施最齐全的服务站,实行家庭医生制,开展"医养结合"项目,提供居家康复、家庭病床、临终关怀等上门服务。而日间照料中心依托专业康复护理组织,可同时为20余位老人提供护理、康复运动等服务,并为社区中度以上的失能失智老人提供包括助餐、助洁、医疗介护等在内的社会化上门安养服务,有助于推进社区居家养老服务。

(三) 老年医疗服务体系特点

1. 医疗机构功能定位相对明确

在养老医疗服务体系中,上海市各级医疗机构功能定位相对明确,提供与之相适应的服务范围。三级医疗机构以治疗性服务为主,提供疑难杂症的治疗,设有老年专科,提供高层次、特需的医疗服务。服务范围辐射全市乃至整个华东地区;二级医疗机构则向辖区内居民提供更为全面的医疗服务,并收治由一级医院、地段医院转诊上来的患者,例如发生并发症、合并症的老年慢性病患者以及慢性转急性患者;社区卫生服务机构则提供预防、保健、医疗、康复、健康教育及计划生育技术指导六位一体的服务,承接大量康复及护理服务,开展老年人的慢性病管理、预防服务工作。同时,通过开展家庭医生签约制度引导患者到基层就诊。目前,社区卫生服务中心收治的患者中,老年人占80%以上。

---

① 虹口曲阳社区打造"一站式"综合为老服务平台[EB/OL]. http://sh.sina.com.cn/zw/h/2016-02-23/detailz-ifxprucs6408601.shtml? from=wap.

王朝昕(同济大学副教授):"现在我们的公立医院定位明确了,这个是值得骄傲的,只是我们供方明确了,但是需方不明确。不过,只要我们自己提供的服务比较明确之后,大家慢慢可以更改过来的。"

2. 为老服务的医疗资源以公立为主,社会资本积极参与

上海市各级公立医疗机构承担了大量老年人医疗和护理服务,政府在老年人医疗服务体系中扮演了主导角色,并通过在综合医院设立老年护理床位、将社区卫生服务机构的床位转为护理床位、将二级综合医院转型为康复医院等举措进一步满足老年人口亟需的护理、康复服务。与此同时,民营资本也积极参与到老年人医疗服务体系的建设中。由于其发展相对灵活,为谋求发展并在为老医疗服务市场上占据较大份额,各类私立医疗服务机构会根据老年人的服务需求及偏好,对服务内容进行调整、完善,以更好地满足老年人的医疗服务需求[①]。2014 年,上海市社会办老年护理院和护理床位占比分别为10.3% 和29.3%,另有 19 家社会办护理站开展居家护理服务[②]。而在养老机构方面,社会办养老机构已成为养老机构发展的重要力量。截至 2014 年底,上海市由社会团体、基金会、企事业单位或个人等社会力量创办的养老机构已达 334 家,养老床位 56 572 张,约占全市养老床位总量的 49.23%[③]。

3. 服务提供方式以老年人口的医疗需求为导向

在政府的引导和支持下,上海市医疗卫生服务体系的发展已对老年人的医疗服务做出一定的倾斜。例如,在社区层面开展重大公共卫生服务项目,其中包括老年人保健,对 65 岁及以上老年人进行健康危险因素调查和一般体格检查,提供疾病预防、自我保健及伤害预防、自救等健康指导;开展家庭医生签约制度,重点针对 60 岁及以上老年人和慢性病患者进行签约,同时家庭医生开设慢性病长处方,解决慢病患者就诊频次高、反复开药的问题;部分社区卫生服务中心开始探索实施"延伸处方",即大医院的药方延伸应用至社区,在社区就能配到大医院的药,免去患病老人为开药而来回奔波,同时减轻了一定的

---

① 张涵,吴炳义,董惠玲.不同类型养老机构老年人医疗服务现状及需求调查[J].中国全科医学,2015(15):1786—1790.

② 数据来源:医疗护理服务体系发展规划(2015—2020 年)(征求意见稿).

③ 数据来源:2014 上海社会福利年报.

费用负担。据统计,2016年,上海市"1+1+1"签约居民共开具延伸处方14.5万张,处方金额达2 870.96万元。由于社区卫生服务中心门诊诊查费减免与药品零差率政策,"延伸处方"药品在社区卫生服务中心开具,居民门诊均次自付平均可减少7.03元[①]。

三、上海市老年人口医疗保障体系现状

(一)上海市医疗保障体系总体架构

上海市医疗保障体系分为托底层、基本层、补充层和自愿层四层(见图2-2)。其中,托底层为医疗救助,基本层包括城镇职工基本医疗保险和城乡居民基本医疗保险两大制度,补充层包括市民社区医疗互助帮困计划、总工会职工互助保障、社区市民综合帮扶等,自愿层包括参保人员自愿购买的商业人寿保险、商业医疗保险等。

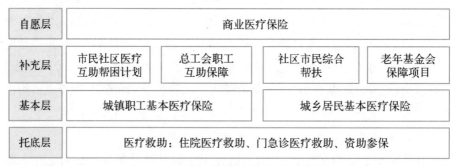

图2-2 上海市医疗保障体系图

(二)上海市医疗保险总体覆盖情况

2015年,上海市三大基本医疗保险包括城镇职工基本医疗保险、城镇居民基本医疗保险和新型农村合作医疗(2016年初与城镇居民基本医疗保险合并为城乡居民基本医疗保险)。其中,城镇职工基本医疗保险参保人数达到1 380.45万人,住院医疗费用中,基金次均支付11 477元,政策范围内住院医疗费用基金支付比例为84.89%;城镇居民基本医疗保险参保272.87万人,住

---

① 上海市卫生计生委."延伸处方"获青睐"社区综改"将深入[EB/OL]. http：//www.wsjsw.gov.cn/wsj/n422/n424/u1ai138193.html.

院基金次均支付 10 551 元,政策范围内住院医疗费用基金支付比例为
75.62%;新型农村合作医疗参保 95.98 万人,政策范围内住院医疗费用基金支
付比例达到 75.02%。在三大基本医保之外,上海市设立了小城镇医疗保险
(针对被征地农民,覆盖 67.98 万人)、市民社区医疗互助帮困计划(覆盖 28.52
万人)等,几类保险合计覆盖人数 1 845.80 万人,常住人口医保覆盖率达到
76.42%。另有红十字会主要管理的少儿住院基金(覆盖 220.11 万人),其中约
1/3 为非户籍儿童,但由于暂时无法与其他医保区分,此处暂未计入。上海市
医疗保险总体覆盖情况如表 2-6 和图 2-3 所示。

表 2-6　2015 年上海市三大基本医疗保险的基本情况

保险类型	覆盖人群	覆盖人数(2015 年,万人)	基金收支(亿元)		待遇水平(2015 年)	
			基金收入	基金支出	住院次均支付(元)	支付比例(%)
城镇职工基本医疗保险	在职职工和离退休人员	1 380.45	750.15	518.94	11 477	84.89
城镇居民基本医疗保险	上海市城镇户口的常住居民(含大学生)	272.87	24.02	26.61	10 551	75.62
新型农村合作医疗	上海市农业户口的常住居民	95.98	20.19	—	—	75.02

数据来源:上海市人力资源与社会保障局网站、2016 年上海统计年鉴。

(三)主要保险制度政策设计

1. 三大基本医疗保险筹资保障制度

三大基本医疗保险筹资保障制度主要为城镇职工基本医疗保险、城乡居民基本医疗保险、小城镇基本医疗保险(镇保)。原新型农村合作医疗于2016 年初已统筹并入原城镇居民基本医疗保险,称为城乡居民基本医疗保险。各项保险制度基本框架如表 2-7 所示。

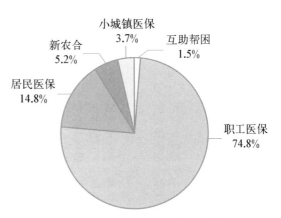

图 2-3　2015 年上海市政府型医疗
保险覆盖人数构成

表 2-7 三大基本医疗保险筹资保障制度一览表

保险类型	覆盖人群	覆盖人数（2014 年）	筹资方式	账户类型	保障范围	待遇水平（2014 年）	行政主管部门
城镇职工基本医疗保险	在职职工和离退休人员	1 353.6 万	单位：8% 个人：2% 附加（单位）：2%	统筹基金、个人账户	门急诊、门诊大病、家庭病床、急诊留观、住院	医疗服务总人次 17 138.27 万 住院医疗费用次均支付 10 670 元 政策范围内住院费用基金支付比例 84.68%	上海市人力资源和社会保障局
城镇居民基本医疗保险（2016 年合并以前）	上海市城镇户口的常住居民（含大学生）	257.66 万				医疗服务总人次 1 658.74 万人次 住院医疗费用次均支付 9 795 元 政策范围内住院费用支付比例 75.55%	上海市人力资源和社会保障局
新型农村合作医疗（2016 年合并以前）	上海市农业户口的常住居民	98.74 万	个人缴费 + 政府补贴	统筹基金	门急诊、家庭病床、急诊留观、住院	医疗服务总人次 1 707.27 万人次 住院医疗费用次均支付 6 349.37 元 政策范围内住院费用基金支付比例 75%	上海市卫生和计划生育委员会
城乡居民基本医疗保险（2016 年合并）	上海市户口常住居民	—				—	上海市人力资源和社会保障局
小城镇基本医疗保险	被征地农民	70.94 万	安置补助费	统筹基金	门急诊、门诊大病、急诊留观、住院	—	上海市人力资源和社会保障局

（1）覆盖人群

城镇职工基本医疗保险针对上海市城镇企业、机关、事业单位、社会团体和民办非企业单位的在职职工和离退休人员。截至 2014 年年末，上海市职工基本医疗保险参保人数达 1 353.57 万人，其中参保职工 946.48 万人，离退休（职）人员 407.09 万人，参加职工基本医疗保险的农民工人数为 284.57 万人。

原新型农村合作医疗与原居民基本医疗保险合并为城乡居民基本医疗保险。覆盖人群包括以下四类：一是具有上海市户籍、年龄超过 18 周岁的人员；二是具有上海市户籍的中小学生和婴幼儿；三是在上海市各高等院校、科研院所中接受普通高等学历教育的全日制本科学生、高职高专学生以及非在职研究生（统称"大学生"）；四是根据实际情况可以参照适用的其他人员。

小城镇保险是一项实行社会统筹和个人账户相结合的社会保险基本制度，包括养老、医疗、失业、生育、工伤等基本社会保险和补充社会保险，而小城镇医疗保险是其中重要一环，参保对象主要是被征地人员，2014 年参保人数约 70.94 万人。

（2）筹资和缴费

城镇职工基本医疗保险基金由统筹基金和个人医疗账户构成。在职职工的缴费基数为本人上一年度月平均工资。本人上一年度月平均工资超过上一年度上海市在职职工月平均工资 300% 的，超过部分不计入缴费基数；低于上一年度上海市在职职工月平均工资 60% 的，以上一年度上海市在职职工月平均工资的 60% 为缴费基数。在职职工个人应当按照其缴费基数 2% 的比例，缴纳基本医疗保险费。退休人员个人不缴纳基本医疗保险费。用人单位的缴费基数为本单位职工缴费基数之和。2016 年起，用人单位应当按照其缴费基数 8% 的比例，缴纳基本医疗保险费，并按照其缴费基数 2% 的比例，缴纳地方附加医疗保险费。在职人员个人缴纳的基本医保费全部计入本人的个人医疗账户；用人单位缴纳的基本医保费的 30% 左右计入个人医疗账户，标准按照不同年龄段有所区别。需要注意的是，退休人员个人不缴纳基本医疗保险费。

城乡居民基本医疗保险资金筹集主要由个人缴费和政府补贴组成，不同年龄段参保人员的筹资标准和个人缴费标准不同。2016 年城乡居民医保基金的筹资标准如表 2-8 所示。

表 2-8   2016 年上海市城乡居民医疗保险筹资标准和个人缴费标准

人 群 分 类	总筹资标准(元)	其中：个人缴费标准(元)	财政补助标准(元)
70 岁以上人员	3 800	340	3 460
60～69 岁人员		500	3 300
19～59 岁人员	2 500	680	1 820
中小学生和婴幼儿	900	100	800

注：2016 年的大学生缴费标准按照中小学生标准执行。

　　小城镇医疗保险筹资渠道由被征地人员的保险费从其安置补助费中一次性支付(不低于 15 年)，筹资和个人缴费标准按照城乡居民基本医疗保险的 50% 确定，2013 年筹资总额 29.89 亿元。

　　(3) 一般保障水平

　　上海市城镇职工基本医疗保险的保险保障水平和保险基金最高支付限额一直在不断提高。自 2016 年 4 月起，上海市城镇职工基本医疗保险基金最高支付限额(简称"封顶线")提高至 42 万元(见表 2-9)。城镇职工基本医疗保险保障门诊急诊、住院、急诊观察室留院观察及门诊大病和家庭病床报销。其中，门诊大病即职工在门诊进行重症尿毒症透析、恶性肿瘤治疗、部分精神病病种治疗所发生的医疗费用，在职职工由统筹基金支付 85%，退休人员由统筹基金支付 92%，其余部分由个人医疗账户历年结余资金支付，仍不足的由职工自负。2014 年，职工基本医疗保险享受医疗服务总人次达 17 138.27 万人次，其中门诊大病和住院为 500.20 万人次；住院医疗费用中，基金次均支付 10 670 元；政策范围内住院医疗费用基金支付比例为 84.68%。

表 2-9   2016 年上海市城镇职工基本医疗保险报销比例

类别	年龄段	门诊急诊报销比例				住院、急诊观察室留院观察报销比例				门诊大病和家庭病床	
		起付标准(元)	超起付标准报销比例			起付标准(元)	最高支付限额(万元)	统筹报销比例	最高支付限额(万元)	统筹报销比例	
			一级	二级	三级					门诊大病	家庭病床
在职职工	44 岁以下	1 500	65%	60%	50%	1 500	42	85%	42	85%	80%
	45 岁以上		75%	70%	60%						

续 表

类别	年龄段		门诊急诊报销比例				住院、急诊观察室留院观察报销比例				门诊大病和家庭病床	
			起付标准（元）	超起付标准报销比例			起付标准（元）	最高支付限额（万元）	统筹报销比例	最高支付限额（万元）	统筹报销比例	
				一级	二级	三级					门诊大病	家庭病床
退休人员	2001年1月1日后	69岁以下	700	80%	75%	70%	1 200	42	92%	42	92%	80%
		70岁以上		85%	80%	75%						
	2000年12月31日前		300	90%	85%	80%	700	42	92%	42	92%	80%
外来从业人员	自2016年4月起享受职工基本医疗保险待遇											

城乡居民基本医疗保险由基金统筹支付，不设个人账户。双保并轨后，城乡居民尤其是农村居民医保待遇进一步提高（见表 2-10）。以往新农合住院费用超过 12 万元不能再结算，而实行城乡统筹后，超过 12 万元的住院费用还可以按照规定比例结算。农村居民各级医院的住院支付比例也有所提高，特别是三级医院的医保支付比例较原来提高 10%～20%，进一步减轻了农村居民到大医院看病的负担。此外，对城乡居民个人负担较重的重症尿毒症透析治疗、肾移植抗排异治疗、恶性肿瘤放化疗、部分精神病治疗等四类疾病的治疗，可由城乡居民大病保险资金按规定再报销 50%。通过以上调整，农村与城镇居民政策范围内住院费用的实际报销水平都超过了 75%。

表 2-10 2016 年城乡居民基本医疗保险报销比例

类型	人群分类	起付标准			医保基金支付比例		
		一级医院	二级医院	三级医院	一级医院	二级医院	三级医院
住院待遇	60岁及以上人员	50元/次	100元/次	300元/次	90%	80%	70%
	60岁以下人员				80%	75%	60%

续 表

类型	人群分类	起付标准			医保基金支付比例		
		一级医院	二级医院	三级医院	一级医院	二级医院	三级医院
门诊待遇	60 岁及以上人员、中小学生和婴幼儿	300 元			70%	60%	50%
	19～59 岁人员	500 元					

注：村卫生室就医不设起付标准。

小城镇医疗保险统筹基金保障门急诊、住院及门诊大病，不设个人账户。2016 年小城镇医疗保险报销比例如表 2-11 所示。自 2016 年 4 月起，上海市小城镇医疗保险基金最高支付限额（简称"封顶线"）提高至 42 万元。"封顶线"以上符合上海市医保规定医疗费用的，仍可报销 80%。

表 2-11　2016 年小城镇基本医疗保险报销比例

人群分类	门诊急诊报销比例				住院、急诊观察室留院观察报销比例			门诊大病	
	起付标准	报销比例			起付标准	最高支付限额（万元）	统筹报销比例	最高支付限额（万元）	统筹报销比例
		一级	二级	三级					
不满 60 周岁	500 元	70%	60%	50%	第一次 1 168 元 第二次 584 元	42	70%	42	70%
60 周岁及以上	300 元								

注：从业人员每次住院、急观所发生的超过起付标准以上部分的医疗费用，由镇保基金支付 70%；按月领取养老金人员每次住院、急观所发生的超过起付标准以上部分的医疗费用，由镇保基金支付 80%；其余部分由参保人员自负。

(4) 对于重大疾病、重点人群的经济风险保护机制

第一，封顶线和起付线的保障设计。对于城镇职工基本医疗保险和小城镇基本医疗保险，"封顶线"以上符合上海市医保规定的医疗费用，仍可报销 80%。

城镇居民基本医疗保险与新型农村合作医疗保险合并成为城乡居民基本医疗保险后，在门诊方面，对农村居民取消了原 5 000 元的封顶线，不设最高支付限额；城镇居民一、二级医院的医保支付比例提高了 5%，19～59 岁

城镇居民的门诊起付标准从原来的 1 000 元下调到 500 元,降低了 500 元。同时,城乡居民在村卫生室就医,不再设起付线,由医保直接按 80% 的比例支付。与合并前相比,无论是城镇居民还是农村居民,门诊费用负担均有所减轻。

第二,城镇职工基本医疗保险综合减负。2004 年,上海市医疗保险局印发《上海市城镇职工基本医疗保险综合减负实施办法》的通知(沪医保〔2004〕126号),对参加上海市城镇职工基本医疗保险的在职职工和退休人员,参保人员年自负医疗费累计超过其年收入一定比例的部分,实施与参保人员年收入挂钩的医疗保险综合减负(以下简称"医保综合减负"),以切实解决部分参保人员自负医疗费的特殊困难。2009 年对适用条件进行调整,具体情况如表 2-12所示。

表 2-12　上海市城镇职工保险综合减负办法

职退状态	年 收 入 标 准	减负方案	
		减负门槛	减负比例
在职	最低生活标准(限患大病或大部分丧劳协保人员,按最低生活标准计算)	25%	90%
	低于最低工资标准的 80%(按最低工资标准的 80% 计算)	25%	
	最低工资标准的 80% 至最低工资标准(按实际收入计算)	25%	
	最低工资标准至社平工资 1.5 倍(按实际收入计算)	30%	
	社平工资 1.5 倍至 3 倍(按实际收入计算)	40%	
退休	低于最低工资标准的 80%(按最低工资标准的 80% 计算)	25%	90%
	最低工资标准的 80% 至最低工资标准(按实际收入计算)	25%	
	年养老金大于最低工资标准(按实际收入计算)	30%	

第三,外来从业人员医保待遇衔接。2016 年 3 月,上海市人力资源和社会保障局发布了《关于 2016 年度外来从业人员参加上海市职工基本医疗保险后医保待遇衔接有关问题的通知》(沪人社医发〔2016〕17 号),针对非城镇户籍外来从业人员(简称"外来从业人员")参加上海市职工基本医疗保险做出了规定:"2016 年 3 月按规定正享受当月外来从业人员医保待遇的人员,自 2016 年4 月 1 日起统一调整为享受职工基本医疗保险待遇;2016 年 3 月新参保的外来从业人员,自 2016 年 4 月 15 日起享受职工基本医疗保险待遇。"这标志着

上海市外来从业人员医保与城镇职工基本医保待遇"全接轨"。

第四，城乡居民大病保险。《上海市城乡居民大病保险试行办法》（沪发改医改〔2014〕2 号）提出对以下四类疾病的治疗予以保障：重症尿毒症透析治疗、肾移植抗排异治疗、恶性肿瘤治疗（化学治疗、内分泌特异治疗、放射治疗、同位素治疗、介入治疗、中医治疗）、部分精神病病种治疗（精神分裂症、中重度抑郁症、躁狂症、强迫症、精神发育迟缓伴发精神障碍、癫痫伴发精神障碍、偏执性精神病）。

2014 年 12 月，上海市卫生和计划生育委员会等发布《上海市新型农村合作医疗商业大病保险实施意见》的通知，提出"罹患上述四类疾病后，在定点医疗机构发生的、符合上海市基本医疗保险报销范围的费用，经新农合基本医疗基金补偿后，参合患者在基本医疗保险政策范围内个人自负的费用，纳入上海市新农合大病保险支付范围，由大病保险基金补偿 50%。不设起付线和封顶线"；此外，设置"按费用"保障方案，对罹患非上述四类疾病的大病患者，住院（含门诊大病）参合农民经新农合基本医疗基金补偿后，当年累计自付政策范围内费用仍超过 1 万元的，对超出部分再补偿 70%，封顶补偿 8 万元。

2015 年 1 月，上海市医疗保险事业管理中心发布《关于上海市城镇居民大病保险委托商业保险机构办理报销的通告》，提出"2015 年 9 月 1 日起，上海市高等院校在校学生患血友病、再生障碍性贫血所发生的医疗费用，一并纳入居民大病保险范围"，"参保居民患上述大病，在上海市基本医疗保险定点医疗机构发生的、符合上海市基本医疗保险规定的个人自负部分，纳入居民大病保险支付范围，由居民大病保险资金报销 50%。其中，参保居民中已参加上海市中小学生、婴幼儿住院医疗互助基金的，应先扣除互助基金支付部分，剩余的自负费用，再由居民大病保险资金报销 50%"。

(5) 老年人筹资与报销情况比较

由上所述，城镇职工基本医疗保障制度的设计对老年人群给予了一定的考虑，按退休状况、年龄分别设立了支付和保障标准，并对年龄较高、退休时间长的人员，分层设计了较低的起付线标准和较高的报销比例。逐步调高最高支付限额的实践，也使医疗费用相对较高的老人群体的利益得到了照顾。同时，城乡居民基本医疗保险也以 60 岁、70 岁为界，分年龄设置了不同的筹资和保障标准，并按医疗机构的级别设置报销和支付比例，与鼓励老年人群向基层医疗机构下沉倾斜的思路一致。

2. 补充医疗保险筹资保障制度

补充医疗保险制度包括市民社区医疗互助帮困计划、总工会职工互助保障、社区市民综合帮扶等，详见表 2-13。

表 2-13　补充医疗保险体系老年人口相关制度设计

保险类型	保障对象	筹资方式	保障范围	保障情况	主管部门
市民社区医疗互助帮困计划	因历史原因，退休回沪人员及其配偶	个人缴费＋政府补助	门诊和住院高额自负医疗费补助	门诊补助 75%～85% 住院补助 50%～60%	市人力资源和社会保障局
市职工互助保障项目	本市职工	个人缴费＋政府补助	综合性帮扶	因项目而异	市总工会
市帮困互助基金会项目	政府制度性救助后仍存在特殊困难群体	政府筹集	综合性帮扶	—	市帮困互助基金会
市老年基金会助医卡项目	本市困难老人	社会募捐	综合性帮扶	500 元助医卡 / 人/年	市老年基金会
市红十字会少儿住院基金	本市儿童	个人缴费＋政府补助	住院和大病门诊	最高支付金额 20 万元，自负部分报销 50%	市红十字会

（1）市民社区医疗互助帮困计划

该计划面向原上海市户籍并由上海市动员分配支援外省市建设，在外省市办理退休（职）手续，享受外省市社会保险待遇，经上海市公安机关批准，报入上海市常住户口的支内、支疆、上山下乡知青、易地安置离退休干部等人员；以及上述人员的外省市户籍配偶中，按照国家有关规定，在外省市办理退休（职）手续，享受外省市社会保险待遇，经上海市公安机关批准，报入上海市常住户口的人员。上海市人力资源和社会保障局发布了《关于做好 2016 年市民社区医疗互助帮困计划有关事项的通知》（沪人社医发〔2015〕42 号），其中规定，2016 年帮困计划资金的筹资标准为 2 740 元，其中参加对象个人缴费 130 元，其余由市、区（县）政府按 1∶1 筹集。门诊医疗互助帮困补贴每人每年 150 元，用于支付门急诊医疗费。社区医疗互助帮困补助报销比例如表 2-14 所示。

表 2-14　社区医疗互助帮困补助报销比例

类　别	门诊高额自负医疗费补助					住院高额自负医疗费补助	
	每年补助（元）	超过每年补助外起付标准（元）	超起付标准补助比例			起付标准（元）	补助比例
			一级	二级	三级		
外省市或原单位有职工基本医疗保险	150	500	85%	80%	75%	按当地标准	60%
外省市或原单位无职工基本医疗保险						1 000	50%

（2）市职工保障互助会

市职工保障互助会坚持自愿性、互助性、公益性原则开展互助互济工作，推行了多项互助保障计划。退休职工住院补充医疗互助保障计划是上海医疗保障体系中一项重要的补充医疗保险。参保人群包括两类：一是单位团体参保，即属于上海市职工基本医疗保险保障范围的退休职工，按自愿原则通过本人原单位的退管会组织团体参保，缴费标准为 252 元／人；二是社区参保，即属于上海市职工基本医疗保险保障范围的社会退休人员等符合社区参保条件的退休职工，缴费标准为 267 元／人。住院、急诊观察室留院观察、家庭病床治疗补充医疗保障金的给付标准是：统筹基金支付范围之内个人自负部分，补偿 60%；统筹基金最高支付限额以上个人自负部分，补偿 70%；门诊大病治疗补充医疗保障金补偿个人自负部分的 50%；在保障期内被保障人的补充医疗保障金，累计最高给付额为 4 万元。该计划自 2001 年推出以来，截至 2016 年 6 月底，累计已为 1 101.22 万人次退休人员支付 60.46 亿元医疗互助保障金。

（3）市帮困互助基金会

市帮困互助基金主要面向特殊困难市民，为其提供应急性、临时性、综合性的帮扶。社区市民综合帮扶是主要项目之一，它的覆盖人群为政府制度性救助后仍然存在特殊困难的对象或政府政策暂时还没有覆盖到的生活困难群体，形式为应急性、综合性的帮扶。社区市民综合帮扶资助资金原则上按照市、区（县）1∶1（或 1∶2）进行筹措和资助。各街镇按照各区（县）的要求筹措相应额度的帮扶资金。资金资助原则上一年一次。截至 2017 年底，上海市民帮困互助基金会在各区县实施的个案帮扶达 6 万余例，实施的"医疗帮困一卡通"等项目帮扶惠及 20 多万人次。

（4）老年基金会

老年基金会向社会各界募集资金，资助老龄事业，帮助困难老人。其资金主要来源于社会捐助。"助医卡"项目针对低保低收入老年人，每人每年发放500元助医卡，可用于定点医疗机构看病就医。2015年，基金会因病个案帮扶总金额达97.78万元。

3. 医疗救助筹资保障体系

医疗救助作为社会救助中的一项专项救助制度，覆盖上海市全体城乡居民，内容包括住院医疗救助、门急诊医疗救助和资助参保。申请医疗救助对象住院治疗、急诊观察室留院观察治疗、门诊大病治疗和家庭病床治疗的基本医疗费用，在扣除基本医疗保险（包括各项减负）等制度性医疗保障给付、各类互助保障形式兑付、家属劳保、商业保险和有关文件规定的单位应承付以及社会互助帮困资助后，仍影响基本生活的，可以提出医疗救助申请。上海市《关于调整和完善上海市医疗救助制度加强住院医疗救助工作的通知》（沪民救发〔2015〕43号）做出如下具体规定：

（1）住院医疗救助

对象范围为：① 无生活来源、无劳动能力又无法定赡养人、扶养人或抚养人的人员，主要是指享受民政部门定期定量救济的孤老、孤儿、孤残等人员；② 上海市城乡低保家庭中的患病住院治疗人员；③ 上海市城乡低收入困难家庭中患病住院治疗人员；④ 市人民政府规定的其他特殊贫困人员；⑤ 散居孤儿。住院医疗救助内容包括住院、急诊观察室留院观察、门诊大病和家庭病床所发生的自负医疗费用。救助标准为：第①、第④类对象，自负医疗费用给予大部或全部救助；第②、第⑤类对象，其自负医疗费用按80%比例给予救助，全年最高救助限额8万元；第③类对象，其自负医疗费用按70%比例给予救助，全年最高救助限额8万元。

（2）门急诊医疗救助

对象范围为：① 上海市城乡最低生活保障家庭成员〔上海市低保家庭中非上海市户籍的家属（配偶、子女）符合"患大病重病、丧失劳动能力、配偶年龄男60周岁、女50周岁及以上、子女未满16周岁或年满16周岁仍在普通中等学校就读"条件的也可以申请〕；② 散居孤儿。其中，享受上海市民政部门定期定量生活补助的特殊救济对象，其自负医疗费用按100%比例给予救助，其他对象按其个人实际自负门急诊医疗费用的50%给予救助；全年累计救助总额不超过600元。

《关于上海市城乡低保家庭成员参加上海市城乡居民基本医疗保险个人缴费及门急诊起付线补助有关事项的通知》（沪民救发〔2015〕46号）对参加居保的低保家庭成员个人缴费部分进行多种形式的补助，并规定"参加居保的城乡低保人员门急诊起付线费用在300元以内的部分，先由个人垫付，在次年第一季度由区县民政部门根据医保部门提供的医疗费信息按实补助"。

（3）资助参保

全额资助低保家庭成员参加红十字会的少儿住院基金；资助低保家庭成员参加居民医保，除就业年龄段不享受粮油帮困的人员需自付120元外，其余人员给予全额资助。

4. 老年护理服务政策

上海市目前正在研究制定长期护理保险制度，在长期护理保险制度出台之前，上海市老年人群的护理需求主要由市民政局的养老服务补贴政策与市人力资源社会保障局(市医保办)的高龄老人医疗护理计划来保障。

（1）养老服务补贴政策

第一，覆盖人群及评估要求。上海市民政局的养老服务补贴政策覆盖人群为60周岁及以上且拥有上海市户籍的老年人。自2004年起，上海市民政局研究建立了养老服务评估机制，并于2013年5月1日起正式实施上海市《老年照护等级评估要求》（DB31/T684—2013，地方标准）。该地方标准依据国际通用的日常生活活动能力（Activities of Daily Living, ADL）量表以及认知功能评估量表，设定了影响老年人日常生活能力的生活自理能力、认知能力、情绪行为、视觉等四大主要模块参数，据此对老年人日常生活能力进行判断，得出"正常""轻度""中度""重度"四种评估结论，以及"轻度""中度""重度"三个照料等级。迄今为止已为近20万老年人提供了相应的评估服务。

第二，筹资来源。2015年8月11日发布的《关于调整上海市养老服务补贴政策有关事项的通知》（沪民老工发〔2015〕7号）中提到，养老服务补贴所需资金纳入财政预算，由市、区两级社会福利彩票公益金出资承担一定额度，其余由市、区县两级财政按1∶1承担。2015年，市、区县两级社会福利彩票公益金各承担6 000万元。

第三，支付标准。对60周岁及以上、低保、低收入且需要生活照料（照料等级分轻度、中度和重度）的上海市户籍老人，给予人均200元/月的居家养老服务补贴。同时设立养老服务专项护理补贴,即在养老服务补贴的基础上,再增加100元/月(中度)、200元/月(重度)的专项护理补贴,根据老年人情况不同,补贴额度也有所区别。2015年居家养老服务补贴情况如表2-15所示。

表2-15 2015年居家养老服务补贴情况

类 别	享受比例	养老服务补贴(元)	养老服务专项护理补贴(叠加,元)		
			轻度	中度	重度
(一)60周岁及以上的低保户籍老人	100%	200	0	100	200
(二)本人及配偶家庭人均收入高于上海市城乡最低生活保障标准、低于上海市城乡低收入家庭标准的户籍老人	80%	200	0	100	200
(三)80周岁及以上、本人月收入高于上海市城乡低收入家庭标准、低于上海市上一年度城镇企业月平均养老金的户籍老人	50%	200	0	100	200
(四)上述(二)、(三)两类中,无子女或90周岁及以上高龄老年人	以上待遇基础上增加20%	200	0	100	200

第四,结算方式。养老服务补贴以非现金的"服务券(卡)"形式,用于兑换各类养老服务,包括:助老服务社等社区居家养老服务组织提供的居家上门照护服务,社区老年人日间服务中心、长者照护之家等社区托养机构提供的养老服务及其他项目化服务。服务内容有生活护理、助餐服务、助浴服务、助洁服务、洗涤服务、助行服务、代办服务、康复辅助、相谈服务、助医服务等10项。

补贴标准根据老年人的照护等级确定,由服务时数及服务单价构成。照护等级为轻度、中度、重度的,月服务时数分别为30小时单位、40小时单位、50小时单位。服务单价逐步统一,以当年度上海市最低小时工资标准为准,并随全市最低小时工资标准的增长逐年同步调整。2015年,照护等级为轻度、中度的服务单价为18元/小时,重度的服务单价为20元/小时。

(2)高龄老人医疗护理计划

第一,覆盖人群及评估要求。《上海市人民政府办公厅转发市人力资源社会保障局等八部门关于上海市开展高龄老人护理保障计划试点工作意见的通知》(沪府办〔2013〕38 号)于 2013 年 6 月 14 日下发,并于 2013 年 7 月在浦东、杨浦、长宁 3 个区的 6 个街镇进行试点运行。该计划依托基本医保制度,对具有上海市户籍、年龄在 80 岁及以上、参加上海市城镇职工基本医疗保险的老人,采用《老年医疗护理服务需求评估调查表》进行评估,经过评估,因疾病、生理功能衰退而达到轻度、中度、重度护理需求等级或患有慢性疾病的独居老年人,给予老年护理费用专项补贴。

2014 年 11 月,新增徐汇、普陀等试点区的 22 个街镇,扩大试点范围至 28 个街镇;2016 年 1 月,将试点范围进一步扩大至全市。2016 年 5 月 1 日起,覆盖人群年龄从 80 周岁及以上下调至 70 周岁以上。

第二,筹资来源。居家医疗护理服务项目纳入基本医疗保险范围,筹资来源与城镇职工基本医疗保险一致。

第三,支付标准。居家医疗护理服务所发生的费用,由城镇职工基本医疗保险统筹基金支付 80%,其余部分由个人医疗账户结余资金支付,不足部分个人自付。对符合民政医疗救助条件的个人,个人自负费用由其居住地所在的区县政府给予 50% 补贴。

第四,结算方式。居家医疗护理服务项目收费标准暂定 50 元/次,今后综合考虑社会经济发展、人力成本和物价变化因素定期做适当调整。每次上门服务时间为 1 小时,经老年医疗护理需求等级评估,照护等级为轻度(限孤老)的,每周上门服务 1 次,中度每周上门服务 2 次,重度每周上门服务 3 次。截至 2016 年 6 月底,累计服务约 15.5 万人次。

5. 商业医疗保险筹资保障体系

商业健康保险作为我国多层次医疗保障体系的重要组成部分,是针对人们高端化、个性化和多样化的医疗需求而建立发展的补充保险制度。我国商业健康险市场中有寿险公司、财险公司(只可经营短期健康险)及专业健康险公司三类主体,销售的产品较全面,覆盖医疗保险、重疾保险、失能保险及长护保险[①]。上海市于 2011 年下发《上海市深化医药卫生体制改革近期重点实施方案》(沪府发〔2011〕18 号),2013 年下发《关于进一步促进上海市社会医疗机构发展实施意见的通知》(沪府办发〔2013〕6 号),鼓励商业健康保险公司与社会医疗机构开展合作。2015 年起,上海市正式尝试将商业保险与大病医保相

---

① 李矛.我国商业健康保险市场发展现状的研究报告——以四大专业健康保险公司为例[D].北京:对外经济贸易大学,2014.

结合,将城镇居民大病保险委托四大保险公司办理①。

目前上海市基本医疗保险体系在覆盖面、筹资水平、保障水平等多方面处于国内领先地位,但从整体来看,上海市商业保险还处于缓慢发展阶段,参与社会基本医疗保障制度建设程度不高,针对老年人群的保险产品不够丰富。目前主要有两种形式:一种是与基本医疗保险相衔接的保险产品,如城乡居民大病保险、城镇职工补充医疗保险,且企业是商业保险最大的投保主体;另外一种是与重大疾病、健康管理、养老等相关的健康保险。根据中国保险统计信息系统数据,截至 2016 年 6 月底,上海市共有 55 家法人保险机构,其中保险集团 1 家,财产险公司 19 家,人身险公司 25 家,再保险公司 3 家,共有 97 家省级保险分支机构,其中财产险分公司 48 家,人身险分公司 47 家。健康险保费收入 109.49 亿元,在上海保险总保费收入中占比为 12.5%,健康险赔款给付 23.85 亿元,占上海保险赔付支出的 8.91%。

从保险方式角度来看,健康保险产品分为疾病保险(约定疾病)、医疗保险(约定医疗行为)、失能收入损失保险(工作能力丧失)和护理保险(生活护理需要);保险期一般分为终身或定期两种,定期的一般设有固定的年限,或约定为自合同成立起至某周岁(60 或 70 周岁)。此处,以中国第一家专业健康保险公司中国人民健康保险股份有限公司和承保上海市城乡居民大病保险的四家保险公司中的中国人寿保险股份有限公司上海市分公司为例,阐述目前商业健康保险的保障情况。

中国人民健康保险股份有限公司医疗保险产品包括针对不同年龄人群的个人医疗保险,有多种保障额度可供选择;疾病保险有关爱健康防癌保障计划、女性特定重大疾病保险、少儿重大疾病保障计划、个人重疾保障计划等,如表 2-16 所示。

表 2-16　人保健康保险计划举例

保险类型	覆盖范围	保险期限	报 销 比 例
关爱健康防癌保障计划	就医绿色通道、肿瘤、身故、护理、老年关爱	投保至 80 周岁	肿瘤 3 万～30 万 住院津贴 300 元/天(最多 100 天) 护理 30 万 身故和老年关爱保费返还(多项享其一)

① 陈珉惺,王力男,杨燕,等.完善上海市基本医疗保险体系研究:基于商业健康保险视角[J].中国卫生政策研究,2015,8(11):52—56.

续 表

保险类型	覆盖范围	保险期限	报 销 比 例
个人重疾保障计划	36 种重疾、8 种特疾、护理、老年关爱	终身	重疾和护理为全部保额 特疾为保额的 30%，(最高 10 万元) 身故和老年关爱为保额的 120%

注：每种保险详情见官网 http://www.picchealth.com/

中国人寿保险股份有限公司是中国最大的寿险公司，提供的产品涵盖生存、养老、疾病、医疗、身故、残疾等多种保障范围。健康保险产品以疾病保障为主，其中一些保障计划还兼具理财功能，如表 2-17 所示。

表 2-17 中国人寿健康保险计划举例

保险类型	覆 盖 范 围	保险期限	报 销 比 例
终身重大疾病保险	40 种重大疾病、10 种特定疾病、身体残疾、身故	出生 28 日至 60 周岁	一次性支付不同金额（6 万～30 万）
住院费用补偿医疗保险	二级及以上医院住院费用	自购买至 70 周岁	视参加医疗保险情况约定合同给付比例

注：每种保险详情见官网 http://www.e-chinalife.com/。

（四）医疗保障体系对老年人口的倾斜政策

1. 医保筹资负担较小

总体来看，三大基本医疗保险在筹资方面对老年人有一定的倾斜。如城镇职工基本医疗保障制度中规定，退休人员个人不必缴纳基本医疗保险费；城乡居民基本医疗保障制度中 60～69 岁、70 岁及以上老年人总筹资标准高于60 岁以下人群，但个人缴费标准分别约为 60 岁以下人群的 70% 和 50%。相对一般人群来说，老年人群的筹资负担相对较小。

2. 医疗费用报销程度较高

首先，从报销来看，老年人群医疗费用报销程度高，体现在两个方面。**一是起付线低**。城镇职工基本医疗保险中，2001 年 1 月 1 日后退休的 60～69 岁、70 岁及以上老年人起付标准低于在职职工的一半，而 2000 年 12 月 31 日前退休的老人起付线为在职职工的 1/5。居保和镇保中，退休人员起付标准也仅为在职职工的2/5。**二是报销比例高**。老年人群超过起付标准，报销比例高于在职职工，其中又以 2000 年 12 月 31 日前退休的老人高于 2001 年 1 月 1 日后退休的 60～69 岁老人，而此类人群又高于 2001 年 1 月 1 日后退休的 70 岁及以上老年人,形成梯度支付。

其次,补充医疗保险和医疗救助中,针对老年人群也有特殊的制度设计。举例来说,市民社区医疗互助帮困计划专门针对原上海市户籍并由上海市动员分配支援外省市建设,在外省市办理退休(职)手续,享受外省市社会保险待遇,报入上海市常住户口的人员,以及老年基金会针对困难老人发放助医卡用作定点医疗机构看病就医等。

第三,上海市医保和民政部门分别按照各自的行政职能设置了老年护理服务政策,向经评估后有需求的户籍老年人提供享受相关护理服务的补贴。如市民政局发放的居家养老服务补贴和专项养老服务补贴,市人力资源和社会保障局给予的老年护理费用专项补贴。

3. 有一定的医疗负担风险防范机制

为了防止灾难性卫生支出的发生,上海市医保体系设置了医疗风险防范机制。**一是封顶线上再报销。**三大基本医疗保险中,城保和镇保在"封顶线"以上的政策范围内的医疗费用仍可报销 80%。**二是综合减负。**对城保参保人员年自负医疗费累计超过其年收入一定比例的部分,实施与其年收入挂钩的综合减负,以切实解决其自负医疗费用负担。**三是针对特殊人群设置大病保险制度予以保障。**包括贫困老人享有医疗救助、城乡居民患重症尿毒症透析治疗、肾移植抗排异治疗、恶性肿瘤治疗及部分精神病病种治疗四类疾病的治疗予以保障。

四、筹资与服务体系存在的问题

(一)管理体制存在条块分割现象,机构之间服务衔接不畅

由于针对老年人的医疗、护理服务分别由卫生和民政两个行政部门管理,同时医疗保障、社区居家护理保障分别由医保和民政两个行政部门管理,衔接不畅、沟通不足,导致差别化待遇。医保仅根据患者所处机构进行支付,造成医疗服务利用的不公平,老年护理服务资源不足和资源浪费的现象同时存在[①]。例如,由于老年护理院有医保支付,获得同样医疗护理服务时,"居住"在老年护理院的老人能够享受医保报销,而居家照护及"居住"在养老机构的老人则无法享受,使老年护理院长期滞留住院现象严重。虽然政府出台了老年照护统一需求评估相关文件,旨在解决此类问题,然而政策出台时间短,尚未

① 彭佳平.上海市老年护理供需现状及对策研究[D].上海:复旦大学,2011.

打破原有体制格局,老年人群需求大,一时之间难以满足。此外,养老机构的医疗照护问题一直没有得到很好的解决,目前上海市共有养老机构661家,其中353家设置医疗机构,其中仅101家进入医保联网结算,占全市养老机构总数的15.3%。老年人难以得到适合自身实际需求的护理服务,也影响了各类老年护理服务的有效利用。

(二)资源配置护理、康复资源总体不足

1. 机构配置有待改善

首先,缺少老年医学统领机构。老年医学学科在医学学科建设中往往处于边缘地带,这一现象在近几年才得到改善。2012年上海市卫生局科教处颁布的"重中之重"临床重点学科建设计划名单中,华东医院老年医学赫然在列,这意味着随着老龄化问题越来越受重视,老年医学学科的发展也渐渐得到市政府的关注。但目前的上海市老年健康服务体系中缺乏一个具有高水平、综合性的老年医学中心作为统领机构,建立老年医学中心可以起到行业带头作用,对越来越多元化的老年人健康服务模式制定标准,并开展人才培训。

其次,护理、康复资源总量不足。在机构配置方面,目前的医疗服务体系以设置医疗机构为主。访谈过程中,专家学者普遍认为现有的医疗资源已经能够满足老年人的医疗服务需求。而各级医疗机构观念上尚不能适应医疗模式的转变,重医疗轻护理,轻视康复服务。而老年人由于其健康状况及需求特点,对护理和康复服务存在大量需求,相对来讲,康复、护理资源显得不足,成为上海市老年医疗服务体系中的短板。此外,资源配置区域分布不均衡,部分郊区的老年护理床位空置,而中心城区一床难求。

　　上海市疾病预防控制中心主任付晨:"康复这一块也是上海一个比较明显的短板,主要的表现是康复机构总量比较少,机构层次也不高。从上海的服务体系来讲,可以有很多在全国乃至世界上比较有名的以治疗为功能的医疗机构,但是没有哪一家康复医院在国际上享有盛誉,在国内也谈不上。我们没有那种非常有品牌的康复医院,这是很明显的一个短板。康复人才更欠缺,另外康复的收费项目也不是很完善。多种因素制约了康复体系的发展。"

2. 部分专业人员短缺

第一，护理评估人员存在短缺。老年人护理需求评估工作需要由有资质的第三方评估人员开展，目前上海市的护理需求评估人员存在短缺。

第二，护理人员缺乏。上海市老年护理服务从业人员存在总体数量不足、流动性大、资质水平不高等问题，与职业化发展的要求还有一定距离。首先，在培训体系方面，医院护工、养老机构护理员、居家养老服务人员三类老年护理服务人员分别归属不同的培训机构，缺乏统一的培训标准、考核标准、鉴定标准和培训机构管理标准，没有与养老护理员的职业等级资格相互衔接的培训体系。其次，老年护理服务由于薪酬水平较低、上升通道狭窄等无法吸引到足够的人才。

第三，家庭医生数量短缺。家庭医生数量短缺导致家庭医生签约制度并没有落到实处。现实的情况是，平均每位家庭医生的签约人数普遍在 1 500～2 500 人之间，工作负荷大，而老年人往往感到签了家庭医生以后却没有享受到相应的服务。究其原因，主要是家庭医生服务范围不清晰、服务动力不足，薪酬制度也有待完善。

> 上海市疾病预防控制中心主任付晨："家庭医生制度，一方面是要完善薪酬制度，要把它变成，这两千个人不是上面给我的任务，而是这一块田就是我承包的。在这种机制下，他才有可能把这个田种好，如果种得好不好和他自己的利益无关，那他就不会好好种这个田了。家庭医生的生产关系还没有转到自己对自己的责任田负责的状态，可能这就是他的激励当中存在的一个问题。"

（三）老年人保障程度较高，但存在保障内容和人群的薄弱环节

首先，保障体系存在空白地带。目前上海市医疗保险体系注重医疗服务项目的覆盖，而忽视护理、康复服务需求。上海市老年人期望寿命长，随着年龄增长，自理能力逐渐下降，照护需求不断增加，更加迫切地需要护理和康复服务保障。由于绝大部分老年护理项目没有纳入医疗保险，目前又缺乏长期护理保险予以保障，护工费用等支出都需要自费，许多老年人难以承受，影响了其护理需求。

其次，**外地常住人口医保异地报销难**。许多外来常住老人没有本地保险。我国医保实行属地管理制度，根据属地的不同，又分别存在着城镇职工基本医疗保险、城乡居民基本医疗保险等医疗保险制度，使异地就医报销更为复杂。相关经办机构、报销目录、报销办法、报销水平均不一致，使得医保信息的共享较为困难。此外，部分地区医保仅为市级统筹，基金统筹层次低，不利于更好地发挥社会保障的互济功能。上海市外来常住老年人口多，且这部分人群中绝大部分异地医保转移接续难，在本地看病就医需要自费，而在外地的医保资金不能使用，造成了资源的巨大浪费。

（四）服务利用方面：浪费与不合理利用并存

1. 无序就医，"照护医院化"和"养老机构化"

目前上海市老年人医疗服务资源较充分，各级机构功能定位也相对明确，虽然近年来已出台各项政策鼓励居民常见病、多发病向基层就诊，但老年人目前仍然以大医院为首选就医机构，对社区卫生服务机构的利用则较低[①]。其原因主要在于两个方面。首先是上海市医疗"一卡通"政策的执行，老年人可以到市内任意一家医疗机构就诊，导致居民患有任何疾病都倾向于到大型三级医院就诊，造成一定程度上的医疗资源浪费，同时也影响到其医疗服务的质量。其次，社区卫生服务机构服务能力有待加强。由于薪酬水平较低、薪酬激励制度不够完善等问题，社区卫生服务机构无法吸引到高层次人才，这些都会阻碍社区卫生服务的健康发展，进而影响到老年人的就医选择。

此外，不少研究发现，老年护理院"压床"现象严重。大量仅需要低层次医疗护理的老年人群选择进入医疗机构养老，甚至有一些老人在医院的老年病区或老年医院享受长期护理服务，利用现有的医疗保险为长期护理付费。也有报道表示，由于医保的作用，老人们认为"地段医院比养老院更实惠"，故想"借"医院床位养老[②]。

2. 过度医疗：老年人服务利用频次高，控费难

老年人医疗服务过度利用情况时有发生。从上海市 65 家社区"1＋1＋1"签约的实时数据来看，2016 年上半年的就诊人次推算到全年为人均 20 多次；

---

① 王荣欣，秦俭，汤哲.我国老年人医疗服务现状及医疗服务需求[J].中国老年学杂志，2011(3)：534—536.

② 许燕君，杨颖华，杨光，等.上海市老年护理床位配置现状及问题[J].中国卫生资源，2014(3)：157—159.

按不同年龄段来看,70～80岁年龄段人均就诊次数达到50多次。我国在经济尚不发达的情况下提前进入老龄社会,属于"未富先老"。医疗费用随着老年人口数量的增长而急剧增长,同时由于劳动力减少,导致医保基金的收入平衡受到严峻的考验。老年人群患病多、药费高,费用难以控制,监管也存在一定困难。

> 上海市人力资源与社会保障局访谈对象:"老年人群医保基金利用是'二八原则',也即80%的医疗费用被老年人消费掉;其他如频次高、药费高、护理费用高等特点也均有。"
>
> 上海市卫生和健康发展研究中心副主任丁汉升:"总体上来说,上海老年人医疗服务供给还是蛮充分的,但在医疗质量方面会产生一定问题。虽然他们能够看病,到处看病,个体、局部的质量可能会高,但是整体质量不一定很好。这个老人今天上午到这个医院去看,下午到那个医院去看,后天到另外一个医院,没有人对他负责,他可能会开很多药,究竟最后吃什么药没人知道,甚至今天开的药跟明天开的药有拮抗作用,那就比较讨厌了。"

3. 护理等服务供不应求

无论通过文献归纳还是专家访谈,"供不应求"俨然已经成为上海市老年医疗护理服务体系中最为严峻且突出的问题[①]。根据《2013年上海市老龄事业发展报告书》的统计数据,上海市为老年人开设的家庭病床有4.97万张,需求量为16.9万张,缺口十分大[②]。从上海市连续6年的老年护理床位数量及构成情况来看,上海市老年医疗护理床位数年增长率(2.42%)远低于老年人口增长速度(4.69%)[③],床位增长严重滞后,出现明显的"供不应求"状况。

4. 部分老年患者医疗费用负担仍然较高

60岁及以上人群的就诊比例特别是住院比例高,造成医疗负担重。2011

① 杨光,杨颖华,许燕君,等.上海市老年护理体系存在的突出问题探索[J].中国卫生资源,2014(3):160—162.

② 郭斌.上海市居家养老医疗服务现状研究[J].潍坊工程职业学院学报,2015(4):67—69.

③ 杨颖华.上海市老年护理服务现状及对策研究[D].上海:复旦大学,2011.

年公立医疗机构出院病人中,39.8%为60岁及以上的患者(而第六次人口普查数据显示,60岁及以上人口占比为15.3%),且41.0%为肿瘤、循环系统疾病。因而,患重病、大病的老年人群医疗负担更重,发生灾难性支出、造成因病致贫的风险较高①。

---

① 李芬,金春林,王力男,等.上海市居民医疗负担有多重?［R］.卫生政策研究进展, 2013.

第 三 章

老年人医疗服务利用及费用现状一览

【导读】

老龄化对政策制定的反应性提出了严峻的要求。上海市是最早进入老龄化的城市之一,上海的现状、问题及相关探索对其他省市都有借鉴意义。本章主要基于 2015 年上海市健康信息网医疗卫生机构数据,全面了解上海市老年人医疗资源消耗分布及费用水平,总结医疗资源消耗特点,结果显示,占总人口不到 20% 的上海市老年人发生的门急诊人次、出院人数分别占全市总量的 60% 和 45%,门急诊费用和住院费用分别占全市总量的 60% 和 50% 以上;与其他人群相比,老年人医疗费用更多流向基层,病种结构主要集中在循环系统、恶性肿瘤、呼吸系统疾病;人均医疗费用随年龄增加整体呈上升趋势,老年人口的住院费用个人负担比例较低。这些数据提示我们,应将老年人口医疗服务利用和医疗费用的特点应用于上海市卫生资源配置规划,更好地满足老年人口医疗服务需求,提高资源的利用效率,为完善卫生筹资制度、建立老年护理保障制度奠定基础。

老龄化程度高、发展速度快是近年来上海市人口结构变化的总体趋势。2004—2015 年,上海市 60 岁及以上户籍老年人口占比从 19.3% 提高到 30.2%。从常住人口看,上海市 2015 年人口抽样调查显示,上海市常住人口中,60 岁及以上、65 岁及以上人口占比分别为 19.49%、12.32%。由于非户籍常住人口快速增长,且其年龄结构较年轻,使得常住人口的老龄化程度和速度趋缓。在医疗保障上,非户籍常住人口与户籍人口一样缴纳医疗保险费,但年轻群体的服务利用次数和医疗费用水平远低于老年人口,可以说,户籍居民享受着非户籍常住人口的"人口红利"。

本章以上海市常住人口为研究对象,旨在分析老年人口的医疗服务利用与费用现状及特点,为探索合理配置倾向于老年人的医疗卫生资源、降低老年人不合理医疗费用的策略、建立有效的医疗费用控制机制提供参考依据。

一、范围界定与分析方法

(一)概念界定

本章将 60 岁及以上界定为老年人口组,将 0～14 岁、15～59 岁分别定义为儿童少年组和中青年组。医疗费用指在上海市各级各类医疗卫生机构发生的费用,包括各级各类医院、社区卫生服务中心、妇幼保健院(所)和专科疾病防治院(所、站)等。

(二)数据来源与方法

数据来源于上海市卫生和计划生育委员会信息中心,门急诊数据出自健康信息网,住院数据出自住院病案首页。本研究中,上海市医疗服务及费用总量数据已剔除外省市来沪就医的份额,为常住人口的统计口径。由于无法统计到外来就医个案,因此机构分布、病种分布、次均医疗费用及医疗费用负担数据为上海市医疗卫生机构全口径,不包含非常住人口。本章主要运用 Excel 和 SPSS 对数据进行采集、处理和分析。

（三）数据处理

健康信息网数据覆盖了所有的公立医院（部队医院除外）、大部分社会办医疗机构，由医院自动上传。2015 年上海市常住人口的门急诊服务利用及费用数据，采用身份证号码匹配的方法，将健康信息网中的身份证号码与公安局常住人口身份证号码库匹配；2015 年，上海市常住人口门急诊人次 2.33 亿人次，门急诊费用 611.84 亿元；样本库门急诊人次 1.27 亿人次，占总量的54.51%；门急诊费用 269.39 亿元，占总量的 44.03%。具体数据如表 3-1 所示。

表 3-1　2015 年上海市门急诊人次和费用样本分布及占比

机 构 类 型	样　本		常住人口		样本占比	
	门急诊（万人次）	门急诊费用（亿元）	门急诊（万人次）	门急诊费用（亿元）	门急诊人次	门急诊费用
医院	5 582.93	171.61	13 733.32	450.15	40.65%	38.12%
社区卫生服务中心	6 968.27	93.14	8 632.98	117.89	80.72%	79.00%
妇幼保健院	104.93	3.07	232.59	6.37	45.11%	48.23%
专科疾病防治院	71.19	1.57	216.50	5.87	32.88%	26.80%
门诊部	—	—	532.37	31.55	—	—
合计	12 727.32	269.39	23 347.76	611.84	54.51%	44.03%

由于样本门急诊数据占比略低，且各类型机构样本数据占比差异略大，因此在分析门急诊服务利用和费用数据时，将样本数据除以样本占总量的比例进行调整，进而推算常住人口的服务量和费用在各个维度的分布结构。针对样本库中缺少门诊部信息，直接采用常住人口的门诊部服务量及费用数据，根据样本社区卫生服务中心门急诊服务量及费用结构予以分摊。以年龄机构为例，具体调整方法如下：

$$\text{某年龄段门急诊人次} = \sum_i \frac{\text{某类机构该年龄段门急诊人次}}{\text{该类机构样本门急诊人次占比}} + \text{门诊部门急诊人次}$$
$$\times \text{社区卫生服务中心该年龄段门急诊人次占比}$$

$$\text{某年龄段门急诊费用} = \sum_i \frac{\text{某类机构该年龄段门急诊费用}}{\text{该类机构样本门急诊费用占比}} + \text{门诊部门急诊费用}$$
$$\times \text{社区卫生服务中心该年龄段门急诊费用占比}$$

i＝医院，社区卫生服务中心，妇幼保健院、专科疾病防治院

$$某年龄段人均门急诊费用 = \frac{某年龄段门急诊费用}{该年龄段常住人口数}$$

住院数据出自住院病案首页,包括住院病案首页中的关键信息,如年龄、性别、就诊机构、住院费用等信息。住院病案首页尚不能区分是否为常住人口,样本住院服务人次 320.12 万人次,占总量(包含外来就医)的 88.41%;住院费用 483.13 亿元,占总量(包含外来就医)的 81.91%。2015 年,上海市常住人口出院人数共计 275.66 万(362.09×76.13%),出院费用 430.67 亿元(589.89×73.01%)。表 3-2 为 2015 年上海市出院人数和费用样本分布及推算情况。

表 3-2　2015 年上海市出院人数和费用样本分布及推算表

机构类型	样本(含外来)		总量(含外来)		样本占比		常住比例	
	出院人数(万人次)	出院费用(亿元)	出院人数(万人次)	出院费用(亿元)	出院人数	出院费用	出院人数	出院费用
医院	304.64	471.55	344.58	574.99	88.41%	82.01%	75.82%	72.57%
社区卫生服务中心	8.33	7.38	9.34	9.62	89.21%	76.64%	94.43%	97.84%
妇幼保健院	7.03	3.99	8.05	4.92	87.36%	81.12%	67.68%	73.56%
专科疾病防治院	0.11	0.27	0.12	0.36	89.84%	76.28%	100%	100%
合计	320.12	483.18	362.09	589.89	88.41%	81.91%	76.13%	73.01%

因样本量占比已超过 80%,本研究对于住院服务量及费用的分析为样本库数据。样本库中包含外来就医服务,在计算全市常住人口的人均住院服务及费用情况时,首先用样本数据除以样本占总量(含外来就医),再乘以常住人口服务量(费用)占比,估算常住人口住院服务总量和费用总量。计算公式如下:

某年龄段人均住院服务量(费用) =

$$\frac{\sum\left(\frac{样本库某类机构该年龄段住院服务量(费用)}{该类机构住院服务量(费用)占总量比例} \times \begin{array}{c}该类机构常住人口住院\\服务量(费用)比例\end{array}\right)}{该年龄段常住人口数}$$

二、医疗资源消耗现状

(一) 人口及医疗资源配置基本情况

2015 年,上海市常住人口共计 2 415.27 万人,其中男性多于女性,占比分别为 51.7%和 48.3%。从年龄构成来看,常住人口主要集中在中青年段,占比达到 71.5%,60 岁及以上老年人占比为 19.5%,65 岁及以上老年人占比为 12.3%。总体看来,上海市已步入老龄化社会,老年人口抚养比(65 岁及以上老年人口数/15~64 岁中青年人口数×100%)达到 15.7%。图 3-1 显示了 2015 年上海市常住人口的年龄情况。

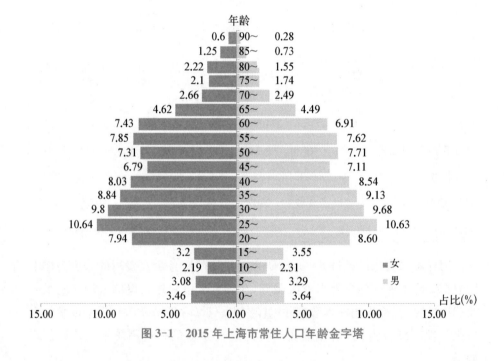

图 3-1 2015 年上海市常住人口年龄金字塔

2015 年,上海市共有医疗卫生机构 5 016 个,其中医院 338 个,占全部机构数的 6.7%。医疗机构共有 12.3 万张床位,其中,分布在医院的比例最高,为 84.3%(见表 3-3)。全市卫生技术人员共计 17.0 万人,其中,医院中的卫生技术人员占比最高,达到了 68.9%;其次是社区卫生服务中心,占比 16.7%(见表 3-4)。

表 3-3　2015 年上海市医疗卫生机构和床位分布

机 构 类 别	机 构 数		床 位 数	
	个	占比(%)	张	占比(%)
医院	338	6.74	103 526	84.30
其中：护理院	25	0.50	6 645	5.41
社区卫生服务中心	1 035	20.63	17 099	13.92
门诊部	633	12.62	—	—
妇幼保健机构	21	0.42	1 317	1.07
专科疾病防治机构	21	0.42	148	0.12
其他	2 968	59.17	723	0.59
合计	5 016	100.00	122 813	100.00

表 3-4　2015 年上海市卫生技术人员分布

机 构 类 别	卫生技术人员		其 中			
	人数	占比(%)	执业(助理)医师(人)	占比(%)	注册护士(人)	占比(%)
医院	117 209	68.87	38 559	61.09	57 911	76.77
其中：护理院	1 835	1.08	368	0.58	593	0.79
社区卫生服务中心	28 498	16.74	12 021	19.05	10 376	13.75
门诊部	8 310	4.88	4 056	6.43	3 262	4.32
妇幼保健机构	2 695	1.58	1 039	1.65	1 280	1.70
专科疾病防治机构	1 107	0.65	564	0.89	374	0.50
其他	12 370	7.27	6 879	10.90	2 235	2.96
合计	170 189	100.00	63 118	100.00	75 438	100.00

(二) 医疗资源消耗分布

1. 年龄分布

2015 年,上海市常住人口门急诊就诊 23 348.70 万人次,其中男性占比为 41.29%,女性占比为 58.71%;出院 275.65 万人,其中男性占比为 46.75%,女性占比为 53.25%。与常住人口年龄构成相比,19.49%的老年人口发生的门急诊人次占总量的 59.95%,出院人数占总量的 45.64%,说明总体上老年人口消耗医疗资源较多。门急诊人次数在各年龄段的分布在 60～64 岁年龄组达到最大值,呈多波峰变化。男性、女性的变化趋势基本一致。出院人数占比随着年龄的变化呈多峰分布，在 40～44 岁年龄组后，住院人数占比急剧升高，在 60～64 岁年龄组达到最大值；随后降低，在 80～84 岁年龄组出现一个小高峰，这与上海市期望寿命年龄基本吻合（总体期望寿命 82.75 岁，男性、女性的期望寿命分别为 80.47 岁、85.09 岁），可能是因为处于临终阶段的人数增加。性别方面，女性在 25～34 岁年龄段的出院人数远高于男性，这与女性的生育高峰期一致。图 3-2 反映了 2015 年上海市各年龄组门急诊和住院服务人次的构成情况。

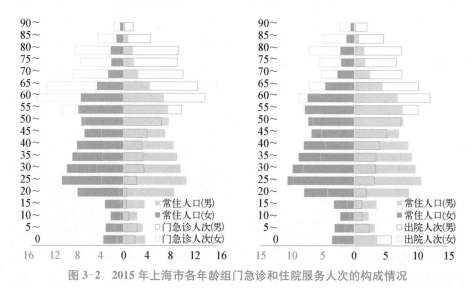

图 3-2　2015 年上海市各年龄组门急诊和住院服务人次的构成情况

　　2015 年，上海市常住人口共发生医疗费用 1 042.61 亿元，其中门急诊费用 611.55 亿元，住院费用 430.30 亿元。费用在各年龄段的分布规律与服务量趋同，但相对于服务量，费用集中度更高，19.49% 的老年人口发生的门急诊费用占总量的 61.22%，住院费用占总量的 52.76%。人口构成与门急诊费用、住院费用及总医疗费用构成相比，50 岁以下费用构成比远低于人口构成比，50～54 岁组两者构成比相近，55 岁以上费用构成比大于人口构成比。图 3-3 反映了 2015 年上海市各年龄组门急诊和住院医疗费用的构成情况。

2. 机构分布

　　不同人群的门急诊服务利用的机构分布有所差异，从不同医疗机构来看，老年人在社区卫生服务中心就诊的比例为 47.04%，明显高于儿童少年组和中青年组，而老年人口组在医院就诊的比例相对较低。从不同医院级别来看，中青年组在三级、二级医院就诊的比例均高于其他两组，老年人口组在三级及二

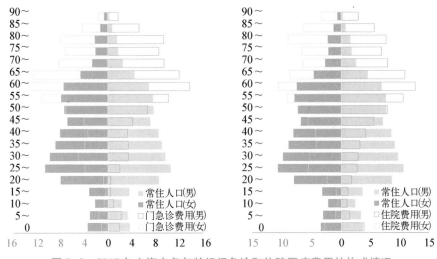

图 3-3 2015 年上海市各年龄组门急诊和住院医疗费用的构成情况

级医院就诊的比例最低,分别为 26.31%,17.80%,而在一级及未定级机构中,老年人口组就诊占比最高,为 5.30%。同样的,不同人群的住院服务利用在不同医疗机构间的分布也有差异。总体来说,全年龄段人口的住院服务利用主要集中在医院。从不同生命阶段来看,老年人口组住院服务利用在医院中的占比为93.78%,低于儿童少年组和中青年组。但是,老年人口组在社区卫生服务中心的住院服务利用占比为 6.08%,明显高于儿童少年组和中青年组。从不同医院级别来看,住院服务利用主要集中在三级医院,而老年人口组在三级和二级医院住院占比相差不大。表 3-5 反映了 2015 年上海市医疗服务利用的机构构成。

表 3-5 2015 年上海市医疗服务利用的机构构成 (单位:%)

机构名称		儿童少年组		中青年组		老年人口组		全年龄段	
		门急诊人次	出院人数	门急诊人次	出院人数	门急诊人次	出院人数	门急诊人次	出院人数
医院		88.96	99.02	71.37	95.08	49.42	93.78	58.82	94.78
级别	三级	58.74	77.22	41.89	63.68	26.31	48.60	33.11	57.81
	二级	29.94	21.80	26.87	31.40	17.80	45.18	21.51	36.97
	一级及未定级	0.28	—	2.61	—	5.30	—	4.21	—

续　表

机构名称	儿童少年组		中青年组		老年人口组		全年龄段	
	门急诊人次	出院人数	门急诊人次	出院人数	门急诊人次	出院人数	门急诊人次	出院人数
其中：护理院	—	0.00	—	0.06	—	1.38	—	0.66
社区卫生服务中心	7.79	0.12	23.20	0.89	47.04	6.08	36.97	3.20
门诊部	0.48	—	1.43	—	2.90	—	2.28	—
妇幼保健院	0.59	0.86	2.65	4.02	0.05	0.06	1.00	1.98
专科疾病防治院	2.18	0.00	1.35	0.01	0.59	0.08	0.93	0.04
合计	100.00	100.00	100.00	100.00	100.00	100.00	100.00	100.00

从各生命阶段的医疗费用机构分布来看，相对于儿童少年组和中青年组，老年人组的医疗费用同样更多地流向社区卫生服务机构及较低级别的医院。门急诊费用中，老年人组流向社区卫生服务机构的构成比（25.98%）分别是儿童少年组和中青年组的 7.38 倍、2.58 倍；流向医院的比例（66.47%）相对儿童少年组和中青年组更低。住院费用中，医院的集中度更高，老年人组流向社区卫生服务机构的比例（3.84%）明显高于儿童少年组和中青年组；流向医院的比例（95.99%）相对儿童少年组和中青年组较低。2015 年上海市住院费用机构构成如表 3-6 所示。

表 3-6　2015 年上海市医疗费用机构构成　　　（单位：%）

机构名称		儿童少年组		中青年组		老年人口组		全年龄段	
		门急诊	住院	门急诊	住院	门急诊	住院	门急诊	住院
医院		93.76	99.63	82.91	97.66	66.47	95.99	73.55	96.89
级别	三级	75.63	89.58	54.00	70.23	37.56	55.56	44.95	63.54
	二级	17.76	10.05	23.97	27.43	19.55	40.43	21.11	33.35
	一级及未定级	0.38	—	4.93	—	9.35	—	7.49	—
其中：护理院		—	0.00	—	0.08	—	1.80	—	0.98
社区卫生服务中心		3.52	0.02	10.08	0.38	25.98	3.84	19.29	2.19

续 表

机构名称	儿童少年组		中青年组		老年人口组		全年龄段	
	门急诊	住院	门急诊	住院	门急诊	住院	门急诊	住院
门诊部	0.94	—	2.70	—	6.95	—	5.16	—
妇幼保健院	0.27	0.35	2.76	1.93	0.04	0.03	1.04	0.84
专科疾病防治院	1.51	0.00	1.55	0.03	0.56	0.14	0.96	0.08
合计	100.00	100.00	100.00	100.00	100.00	100.00	100.00	100.00

3. 病种分布

根据数据库结构,只能在住院服务中区分出病种,根据 ICD-10 编码将疾病归类为 21 种。就上海市 2015 年的数据来看,不同生命阶段对住院医疗服务利用情况在不同病种间的占比分布存在差异。儿童少年组中,出院人数占比最高的前五种疾病分别是呼吸系统疾病(27.66%)、先天性疾病(11.72%)、新生儿疾病(11.40%)、其他疾病或医疗服务(6.00%)、神经系统疾病(5.90%);中青年组中,出院人数占比最高的前五种疾病分别是妊娠分娩和产褥疾病(17.67%)、其他疾病或医疗服务(13.90%)、泌尿系统疾病(9.40%)、恶性肿瘤(9.34%)、消化系统疾病(8.80%);老年人组中,出院人数占比最高的前五种疾病分别是循环系统疾病(27.97%)、恶性肿瘤(11.72%)、呼吸系统疾病(11.19%)、其他疾病或医疗服务(10.06%)、消化系统疾病(8.50%)。由此可见,老年人口组对住院医疗服务利用前三的病种合计占比超过 50%,与本市老年人疾病谱特点相对一致。

21 种疾病的住院费用在儿童少年组、中青年组和老年人口组的占比分别为 5.34%、41.90% 和 52.76%。儿童少年组中,住院费用占比最高的前五种疾病分别是先天性疾病(26.96%)、呼吸系统疾病(10.64%)、新生儿疾病(8.86%)、恶性肿瘤(6.53%)、神经系统疾病(6.45%);中青年组中,住院费用占比最高的前五种疾病分别是恶性肿瘤(17.29%)、循环系统疾病(11.93%)、损伤和中毒(11.55%)、其他疾病或医疗服务(9.64%)、消化系统疾病(8.25%);老年人组中,住院费用占比最高的前五种疾病分别是循环系统疾病(31.98%)、恶性肿瘤(16.38%)、呼吸系统疾病(9.97%)、消化系统疾病(6.91%)、损伤和中毒(6.83%)。结合出院人数集中度来看,儿童少年组中,服务利用排名第二的先天性疾病负担最重;中青年组中,服务利用排名前三的疾病(妊娠分娩和产褥疾病、其他疾病或医疗服务和泌尿系统疾病)发生的住院医疗费用不高，反倒是恶性肿瘤负担更重；老年人口组中，住院医疗费用排序与服务利用排序则相对一致，服务利用排名前三的病种（循环系统、恶性肿瘤和呼吸系统疾病）住院费用占比达到 58.33%。

4. 费用类型分布

从不同年龄段来看，儿童少年组、中青年组、老年人口组费用类型占比中均是药费占比最高，手术材料费用占比最低。横向比较来看，老年人门急诊和住院药费占比均高于其他两组，分别达到 73.52% 和 38.70%。相比之下，老年人劳务性费用比例则相对较低，门急诊劳务性费用占比仅为 9.61%，住院劳务性（综合医疗服务＋治疗）费用占比为 18.73%，远低于其他两组。2015 年上海市门急诊和住院医疗服务费用类型构成如图 3-4、图 3-5 所示。

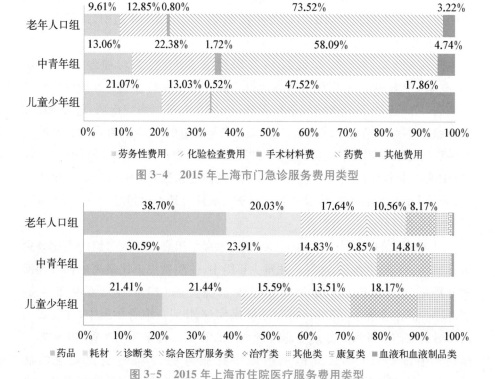

图 3-4　2015 年上海市门急诊服务费用类型

图 3-5　2015 年上海市住院医疗服务费用类型

（三）医疗资源消耗水平及负担

1. 次均医疗费用

2015 年，上海市常住居民次均门急诊费用为 262.01 元，次均住院费用为

15 630.99 元。各年龄组门急诊次均医疗费用呈波动变化,60～79 岁老人的次均门急诊费用处于较低水平;80 岁以后,男性的次均费用增加,女性持平。老年人口中,男性的次均费用高于女性(见图3-6)。次均住院费用中,中青年组较低,老年人口各年龄段总体较高,且呈逐步上升趋势。性别之间比较,各年龄段男性的次均住院费用均高于女性(见图 3-7)。

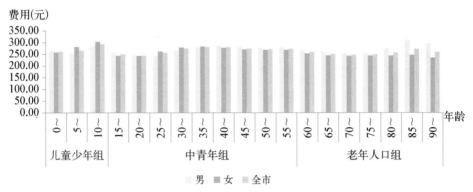

图 3-6　2015 年上海市各年龄组门急诊次均费用水平

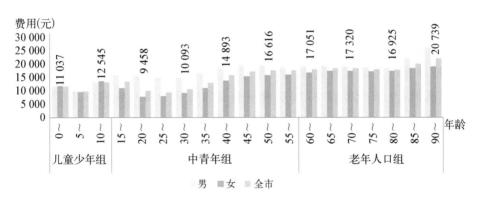

图 3-7　2015 年上海市各年龄组次均住院费用水平

从医疗机构类别来看,医院的医疗服务次均门急诊和住院费用均明显高于其他机构。从不同医院级别来看,一级及未定级机构次均门急诊费用高于其他级别,三级医院次均住院费用高于其他级别,且老年人口组次均门急诊和住院费用普遍高于中青年组和儿童少年组。值得一提的是,老年人口组在社区的次均门急诊费用虽然高于其他组别,但相差不大,而住院次均费用则远高于社区其他组别水平,达到 11 402.19 元。表 3-7 反映了 2015 年上海市不同医疗机构次均医疗费用的情况。

表 3-7　2015 年上海市不同医疗机构次均医疗费用　（单位：元）

机构名称		儿童少年组		中青年组		老年人口组		全年龄段	
		门急诊	住院	门急诊	住院	门急诊	住院	门急诊	住院
医院		277.56	11 197.83	310.86	14 328.05	347.62	18 478.70	327.50	15 957.29
级别	三级	339.03	12 916.90	344.95	15 436.37	368.95	20 608.37	355.61	17 168.51
	二级	156.22	5 130.72	238.75	12 227.98	283.91	16 134.87	257.08	14 093.44
	一级及未定级	354.16	—	506.44	—	455.70	—	466.42	—
其中：护理院		—	0.00	—	19 688.63	—	23 564.76	—	23 401.45
社区卫生服务中心		118.94	1 901.76	116.31	6 054.66	142.77	11 402.19	136.64	10 679.85
门诊部		515.45	—	504.37	—	619.24	—	592.63	—
妇幼保健院		120.47	4 530.94	279.51	6 681.20	204.19	8 774.69	273.46	6 641.55
专科疾病防治院		182.26	0.00	306.75	23 989.82	245.16	30 694.22	271.41	29 596.36
合计		263.34	11 129.33	267.61	13 948.73	258.46	18 052.29	261.92	15 610.28

从不同病种来看，次均住院费用因病种不同而有差异。老年人口组中，精神和行为障碍疾病次均费用达到 4.24 万元，为所有组别所有疾病的最高值；儿童少年组中，次均费用最高的疾病为耳科疾病（3.87 万元）；中青年组中，次均费用最高的疾病为损伤和中毒（2.62 万元）（见图 3-8）。

2. 人均医疗费用

2015 年，上海市常住人口人均医疗费用为 4 421.39 元，其中人均门急诊费用为 2 533.21 元，人均住院费用为 1 888.18 元。总体来看，人均医疗费用随着年龄增加整体呈上升趋势，其中人均门急诊费用在 45 岁以后显著升高，在 80～84 岁年龄组达到最大值，随后有所降低；人均住院费用在 0～4 岁组较高，随后降低，在 5～44 岁年龄阶段变化较平缓，在 60 岁以后，人均住院费用急剧增高。综合门急诊和住院费用来看，85～89 岁老年人人均医疗费用最高（2.32 万元），90 岁以上老年人门急诊费用略有下降，住院费用一直上升。图 3-9 反映了 2015 年上海市各年龄段人均门急诊及住院费用。

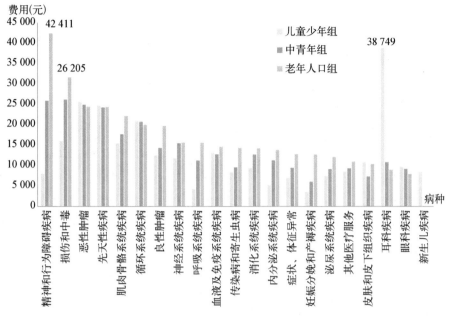

图 3-8　2015 年上海市不同病种次均住院费用

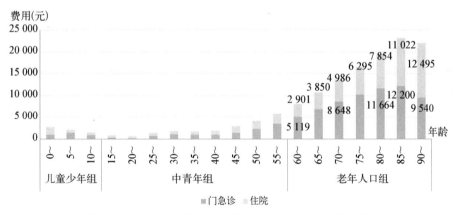

图 3-9　2015 年上海市各年龄段人均门急诊及住院费用

3. 医疗费用负担

从不同医疗机构来看,医院住院患者的个人负担比例高于社区卫生服务中心和专科疾病防治所,低于妇幼保健院。从不同医院级别来看,三级医院的自付比例高于二级医院。从不同医院类别来看,护理院的住院费用自付比例较低。从不同生命阶段来看,老年人口组的住院费用个人负担比例较低(见表 3-8)。

表 3-8　2015 年上海市不同医疗机构住院费用负担　（单位：%）

医疗机构		儿童少年组		中青年组		老年人口组		全年龄段	
		自负比例	自付比例	自负比例	自付比例	自负比例	自付比例	自负比例	自付比例
医院		33.81	64.53	34.33	53.21	24.10	37.25	28.96	45.59
级别	三级	34.51	65.75	37.31	57.44	29.29	45.91	33.40	52.71
	二级	27.61	50.92	26.73	42.96	16.94	25.39	20.49	20.50
其中：护理院		—	—	4.76	6.46	4.45	6.69	4.47	6.68
社区卫生服务中心		35.51	45.77	19.28	21.88	9.93	11.09	10.63	11.90
妇幼保健院		76.25	98.44	38.76	73.74	30.50	48.69	39.44	73.96
专科疾病防治所		—	—	14.20	21.40	12.56	19.09	12.77	19.40
合计		33.96	64.68	34.37	53.54	23.71	36.51	28.75	45.20

注：自负比例是指医保范围内个人自负费用占医保范围内所有费用比例，自付比例是指医保范围内自负和医保范围外自费费用之和占总医疗费用比例，下同。

不同生命阶段的负担型病种有所不同。根据疾病住院次均费用由高到低排序，得到不同生命阶段对应的前十位病种。其中老年人精神和行为障碍疾病、损伤和中毒、恶性肿瘤的次均费用占据前三，住院次均费用分别为 4.24 万元、3.16 万元、2.44 万元，恶性肿瘤自负费用占比高达 35.75%（见表 3-9）。

三、老年人医疗资源消耗特点

（一）老年人利用了更多的医疗服务，花费了更多的医疗费用

从总量结构看，全市医疗服务利用与费用总体趋势随着年龄的增加而增长，并在 60～64 岁年龄组达到峰值，且在不同年龄段的老年人中呈现逐步下降的趋势，在 80～84 岁组有局部小波峰。老年人门急诊、住院医疗费用占全部医疗费用比例分别超过了 60% 和 50%，且集中在 60～64 岁、80～84 岁年龄组，人均医疗费用是儿童少年组、中青年组的 4 倍以上，说明上海市老年人消耗了更多的医疗资源。

从上海市医疗保险统计数据来看，2015 年门急诊、住院就诊人数均在 60～64 岁达到高峰后开始下降，并在 80 岁出现局部峰值，其中，60～64 岁老

表 3-9 2015 年上海市次均住院费用前十的病种的负担情况

排名	儿童少年组				中青年组				老年人口组				全年龄段			
	病种	次均费用（万元/次）	自负比例（%）	自付比例（%）	病种	次均费用（万元/次）	自负比例（%）	自付比例（%）	病种	次均费用（万元/次）	自负比例（%）	自付比例（%）	病种	次均费用（万元/次）	自负比例（%）	自付比例（%）
1	耳科疾病	3.87	71.35	93.30	损伤和中毒	2.62	35.53	64.19	精神和行为障碍疾病	4.24	14.99	20.16	精神和行为障碍疾病	2.99	15.22	28.23
2	恶性肿瘤	2.56	31.00	61.33	精神和行为障碍疾病	2.59	15.98	35.91	损伤和中毒	3.16	23.05	51.10	损伤和中毒	2.75	30.34	58.81
3	先天性疾病	2.47	28.60	59.70	恶性肿瘤	2.50	44.86	64.68	恶性肿瘤	2.44	35.75	55.50	恶性肿瘤	2.47	39.73	59.66
4	循环系统疾病	2.08	25.18	51.08	先天性疾病	2.43	37.07	58.88	先天性疾病	2.44	26.58	47.30	先天性疾病	2.46	31	58.48
5	损伤和中毒	1.60	33.10	64.10	循环系统疾病	2.07	25.10	40.68	肌肉骨骼系统疾病	2.21	26.64	51.90	循环系统疾病	2.02	20.74	31.05
6	肌肉骨骼系统疾病	1.54	42.25	77.53	肌肉骨骼系统疾病	1.77	34.11	57.28	循环系统疾病	2.00	19.41	27.99	肌肉骨骼系统疾病	1.95	30.77	55.34
7	血液及免疫系统疾病	1.31	38.49	66.35	神经系统疾病	1.55	35.15	53.25	良性肿瘤	1.97	33.93	50.20	良性肿瘤	1.50	38.85	57.13
8	良性肿瘤	1.25	54.39	86.04	良性肿瘤	1.43	38.97	56.71	神经系统疾病	1.56	19.54	30.49	神经系统疾病	1.48	26.69	43.90
9	神经系统疾病	1.18	32.40	69.29	血液及免疫系统疾病	1.28	34.98	50.60	呼吸系统疾病	1.56	19.27	25.44	血液及免疫系统疾病	1.35	30.38	46.36
10	皮肤和皮下组织疾病	1.08	69.05	99.00	消化系统疾病	1.27	31.5	44.37	血液及免疫系统疾病	1.46	21.04	30.04	消化系统疾病	1.32	27.45	39.89
合计		1.90	34.39	65.65		1.97	35.27	55.10		2.08	23.93	37.60		2.02	29.19	46.58

年人门急诊就诊人次占比（13.9%）是 0～19 岁组（6.0%）的两倍多，且医疗费用也集中在 60～80 岁的年龄阶段；60 岁及以上老人两周患病率是全人群的 2.4 倍；慢性病年患病率是全人群的 1.8 倍；老年人两周就诊率、年住院率分别为 44.49%、12.14%，远高于全人群的平均水平（21.91%、6.69%）。本次样本数据分析结果与上海市老年人口整体医疗服务利用、医疗费用特征一致。

（二）相对而言，老年人倾向于更多地利用基层医疗服务

从全市医疗费用机构分布来看，门急诊 70%、住院 90% 以上的医疗费用发生在医院，但与儿童少年组和中青年组相比，老年人在社区卫生服务中心的门急诊医疗费用占到了 27.9%，是儿童少年组和中青年组的 9 倍和 2 倍，84 岁以上老年人在社区卫生服务中心的住院医疗费用占比最高。从趋势来看，老年人医疗费用表现出不断流向二级及以下医疗卫生机构特别是社区卫生服务中心的趋势，社区卫生服务中心、二级医院、护理院费用占比明显升高，这与 2013 第五次国家卫生服务调查分析报告以及蒋艳等（2016）[1]学者的研究结果相一致，老年人就医流向趋于合理。

近年来，上海市以社区卫生服务中心为平台推行家庭医生制度，以老年人为重点签约对象，针对老年人的医疗、康复、护理、临终关怀等多方面需求提供全程服务。从老年人医疗服务利用和费用特征来看，老年人对社区卫生服务中心等基层医疗卫生机构的利用程度更高，更方便与家庭医生建立稳定持久的社会关系，充分发挥基层的作用，保障老年人的健康。

（三）老年人医疗支出以药品为主，财务风险基本得到保护

从费用结构上看，药品费用支出是老年人最主要的医疗费用支出，本次调查显示，老年人口组门急诊、住院药品费用占比最高，分别为 73.5% 和 38.7%，其次是门诊化验检查费用（12.8%）、住院耗材费用（20.0%）和诊断费用（17.6%）。本结果与 2015 年上海市医保统计数据分布趋势相似（其门急诊药费占比 70%、化验费 10%、检查费 7%，住院药费占比 38%、化验费 13%、检查

---

① 蒋艳，赵丽颖，满晓玮，等.2002—2014 年北京市卫生总费用医疗机构费用及药品费用流向分析[J].中国卫生经济，2016，35（5）：45—47.

费 6%）；与全国情况（药品费用占门诊和住院费用的比例分别为 52%、43%）相比，上海市门诊药费占比偏高，也高出其他国家 10%～20% 的平均水平[1][2]。2015 年，出院人数占比最高的前三种疾病分别是循环系统疾病、恶性肿瘤和呼吸系统疾病，这也是住院费用占比最高的前三种疾病，而药品费用占比较高的疾病前三位中包括了呼吸系统疾病和恶性肿瘤。这与老年人疾病特点相吻合。

2015 年上海市老年人门急诊人均费用是少年儿童组和中青年组的 8.2 倍、6.7 倍，次均费用是 1.6 倍和 1.3 倍。从不同年龄段老年人费用负担来看，随着年龄增长，老年人人均门急诊费用在 85～89 岁达到顶峰，住院费用呈不断上升趋势，这与老年人终末期费用支出较大有关；老年人医疗费用医疗保险报销比例总体维持在 60% 以上，远高于少年儿童组和中青年组，体现了上海市医疗保险体系对老年人的倾斜政策，老年人的筹资和自付负担相对较小，但与上海市医保统计数据相比（其门急诊报销比例 78.3%、住院报销比例 83.4%）还存在较大差距。

（四）部分老年人仍存在较重就医负担，护理康复需求待进一步保障

结合次均费用水平看老年人个人负担绝对值，以恶性肿瘤为例，2015 年上海市老年人次均费用 2.44 万元，医保范围内自负比例 35.7%，自付比例 61.3%，每个老年人需自行承担 1.50 万元。部分恶性肿瘤后期需要自费药品维持治疗，进一步加重了老年人的负担。而从商业保险发展现状看，目前针对老年人的商业医疗保险市场规模较小，但其自付比例远低于其他保险（2015 年上海市老年人口组住院自负比例仅为 4.9%），亟待进一步发挥商业医疗保险的补充作用，提高老年人的医疗保障水平。

此外，老年人因为失能和残障发生率大，生活不能自理的比例也在升高，对护理及康复服务需求较大，多个研究显示，不同费用之间具有替代作用，舒缓疗护费用的增加伴随着住院费用及其他类型医疗费用的降低，医院的舒缓疗护类咨询有助于节省 9%～25% 的费用，越早进入舒缓疗护环节，节省的费

---

① 董国蕊,陈丽.医院药品费用占比的分析与调控[J].现代药物与临床,2012,27(6)：602—605.

② 牟蘋.综合医院药品费用分析与政策研究[D].北京：北京中医药大学,2010.

用越多①②③，如若排除护理费用，医疗费用随着死亡年龄的增长而减少④。从本次研究数据结果看，尽管老年人口组康复类型费用占比比其他生命阶段高，但也只占到1.1%，在护理院的次均医疗费用是在社区卫生服务中心的两倍多，也高于在三级医院的次均医疗费用，老年人护理费用负担较重。在我国老年人口医疗费用急剧上涨、医保筹资压力不断增大的背景下，建立老年人护理保障制度有助于缓解综合医院的就诊压力。

实际上，我国部分地区已经加快了老年护理保险建设步伐，山东省青岛市在2012年开始着手建立长期医疗护理保险制度，2015年出台《青岛市长期医疗护理保险管理办法》(青人社发〔2014〕23号)，创新开展医疗专护、护理院医疗护理、居家医疗护理和社区巡护等多种服务形式，失能患者在家或养老机构就能得到医疗护理，老人及家属医疗负担大大减少⑤，上海市2017年起试点推行长期护理保险制度，相关效果待进一步评估。

四、局限与不足

受限于数据可得性和质量，本章仅对卫生计生统计部门收集的医疗机构内部发生的医疗费用进行分析，未将在医疗机构外部发生的购药行为等考虑在内，且部分机构，如部队驻沪医院、村卫生室和诊所等，未纳入统计口径对全市医疗费用的影响大致在10%以内(2015年，几类机构总收入占所有发生医疗费用机构总收入的比例为8.19%)。在对常住人口住院医疗服务利用和医

---

① May P, Garrido M M, Cassel J B, et al. Prospective cohort study of hospital palliative care teams for inpatients with advanced cancer: Earlier consultation is associated with larger cost-saving effect[J]. Journal of Clinical Oncology, 2015, 33(25): 2745—2752.

② Kerr C W, Donohue K A, Tangeman J C, et al. Cost savings and enhanced hospice enrollment with a home-based palliative care program implemented as a hospice-private payer partnership[J]. Journal of palliative medicine, 2014, 17(12): 1328—1335.

③ McCarthy I M, Robinson C, Huq S, et al. Cost savings from palliative care teams and guidance for a financially viable palliative care program[J]. Health services research, 2015, 50(1): 217—236.

④ Temkingreener H, Meiners M R, Petty E A, et al. The use and cost of health services prior to death: A comparison of the Medicare-only and the Medicare-Medicaid elderly populations.[J]. Milbank Quarterly, 1992, 70(4): 679—701.

⑤ 袁彩霞.我国老年长期护理保险制度实施路径研究[D].南京：南京师范大学，2014.

疗费用进行匡算时,由于外来就医数据不能细分到年龄别,本章假设外来就医人群均是根据病情需求选择来沪就医,因此仅用各机构的总体外来就医比例对常住人口进行推算,默认常住人口和外来就医人群不存在年龄别差异。此外,目前本章仅针对2015年上海市截面数据进行分析,随着老龄化程度的加深、老年医学中心的建成、老年护理保障制度等政策的出台,上海市老年人医疗服务利用和费用的变化趋势有待进一步研究。

第四章

终生医疗费用模型及启示

【导读】

　　国内外经验均表明,老年人群医疗费用高于其他年龄人群。本研究基于上海市医疗大数据,以 2015 年全市常住人口全年龄段医疗服务利用和医疗费用的横截面数据,利用现时寿命表模拟终身医疗费用。结果显示,60~64 岁组尚存者人均余生期望医疗费用占人均终生医疗费用的比值,门急诊为 77.46%,住院为 72.93%,总医疗费用为 75.56%。此外,90 岁以上组尚存者人均余生期望总医疗费用占人均终生总医疗费用比值也达 22.90%。与国际上类似研究相比,上海市老年人群的医疗费用在终生费用中的比例较高,且具有 80 岁及以上老年人群医疗费用预期主要流向住院、80 岁以下老年人群医疗费用预期主要流向门诊的特征。建议推进就医、养老进一步下沉社区,充分调动利用社区资源;试行长期护理保险制度,促进老年照护公共服务供给;控制住院费用,引导优化医疗费用使用结构。

多项研究表明，老年人口人均医疗费用及其增长速度高于其他年龄组[1][2]，原因是随着年龄增加，健康状况下降，医疗服务需求和费用增加[3][4]。Alemayehu 等（2004）[5]采用现时寿命表和横截面医疗费用数据模拟终身医疗费用，结果显示，平均约 1/3 的医疗费用发生在 40～64 岁；65 岁及以上的医疗费用占终身医疗费用的 1/2；对于 85 岁及以上的老年人，期望医疗费用占据终身医疗费用 1/3 以上。国内大多数研究发现，随着年龄的增加，对医疗服务的需求会随之增加。许多学者发现，老年人口医疗费用比其他年龄组高。一些研究认为，老年人口对医疗服务需求较高，因而随着老龄化程度加深，医疗费用将快速增加[6]，但也有研究认为医疗费用增长受多重因素影响，年龄结构变化有影响但没有其他因素的影响大[7][8][9][10]，可能影响医疗费用增长的因素包括性别、年龄、婚姻状况、城乡身份等。

关于老龄化与医疗费用关系的研究主要集中在两个方面。

一是老年人口与其他年龄组平均医疗费用的比较研究，包括横断面研究和队列研究。老年人口的平均医疗费用普遍高于其他年龄组，费用增长速度

① Culter D M，Meara E. The medical costs of the young and old：A forty-year perspective[M]. Chicago：University of Chicago Press. 1998：215—246.

② Reinhardt U E.Does the aging of the population really drive the demand for health care？[J]. Health Affairs（Millwood），2003，22：27—39.

③ Waldo D R，Lazenby H C.Demographic characteristics and health care use and expenditures by the aged in the United States：1977—1984[J].Health Care Financing Review，1984，6：1—29.

④ Buchner F，Wasem，J.“Steeping” health expenditure profiles[J]. Geneva Papers on Risk & Insurance Issues & Practice，2006，31(4)：581—589.

⑤ Alemayehu B，Warner K E.The lifetime distribution of health care costs[J]. Health Serv Res，2004，39：627—642.

⑥ 黄婷婷. 我国人口老龄化对卫生总费用增长的影响[D]. 厦门：厦门大学，2012.

⑦ 王超群. 老龄化是卫生费用增长的决定性因素吗？[J]. 人口与经济，2014（3）：23—30.

⑧ 马爱霞，许扬扬. 我国老年人医疗卫生支出影响因素研究[J]. 中国卫生政策研究. 2015（7）：68—73.

⑨ 余央央. 老龄化对中国医疗费用的影响——城乡差异的视角[J].世界经济文汇. 2011（5）：64—78.

⑩ 上海市人民政府. 市政府关于印发《上海市长期护理保险试点办法》的通知(沪府发〔2016〕110 号).

也相对较快。但居家护理和社区护理的发展对医疗服务的替代作用，降低了老年人口的总体医疗费用水平。从中可推断，服务体系结构是医疗费用的重要影响因素，将影响老龄化实际产生的作用。

二是分析年龄与其他影响因素变化的情况下，老龄化对医疗费用的影响。对医疗费用影响较大的因素包括收入提高、参保人数增加、医疗技术进步等，除少数研究认为老龄化对医疗费用的影响为负或不相关，普遍认为年龄结构变化对医疗费用的归因贡献度不一。

随着信息系统的发展，医疗大数据逐渐形成，挖掘信息服务于政策制定是当务之急。上海是我国最早进入老龄化的地区之一，在信息化建设方面处于全国前列，开展全样本研究的基础较好。本研究基于大数据，全面了解上海市常住人口医疗服务利用和医疗费用的数量和构成。将医疗费用数据与生命表模型结合，模拟终身医疗费用，探索医疗费用随年龄增长的变化规律，预测医疗费用随着老龄化程度加深而变化的情况，为完善卫生筹资制度、建立老年护理保障制度提供本土研究证据。

一、终生医疗费用模型及其测算方法

医疗费用数据同本书第三章，2015 年上海市全人口现时寿命表数据（以 5 岁为组距）来自上海市疾病预防控制中心。利用现时寿命表和横截面医疗费用数据模拟终身医疗费用，假定技术、价格和其他影响卫生服务成本的因素保持恒定，疾病的患病率、发病率、发展进程、医疗服务成本都不随时间变化，那么可用年度医疗费用的年龄分布反映医疗费用在患者终生的分布情况。该方法的优点是剔除了医疗服务价格、医疗技术进步等混杂因素的影响。

在终生医疗费用模型中，余生医疗费用为个体在剩余的寿命中医疗费用的总和。人均余生医疗费用的计算方法如下：

① 按出生时计算的某年龄人均余生期望医疗费用（LECB, lifetime expected cost at birth），是将队列在该年龄时的余生期望医疗费用除以最初的队列样本量。

假设：C_x＝分年龄组的人均医疗费用（$x＝0\sim,1\sim, 5\sim, 10\sim,\cdots,90\sim$；90 岁以上合并为一个年龄组，以下同），$L_x$＝在年龄组的队列存活人年数，$l_0$＝0 岁时的存活人数（初始队列人数），那么，在 x 岁时按出生时计算的某年龄人均余生期望医疗费用：$\text{LECB}_a = \sum\limits_{x=a}^{95}\left(\dfrac{C_x L_x}{l_0}\right)$；在 x 岁时某年龄人均余生期望医疗费用占人均终生期望医疗费用比值：$\text{RLECB}_a = \text{LECB}_a / \text{LECB}_0 = \sum\limits_{x=a}^{95}\left(\dfrac{C_x L_x}{l_0}\right) \bigg/ \sum\limits_{x=0}^{95}\left(\dfrac{C_x L_x}{l_0}\right)$。

② 存活到某年龄的人均余生期望医疗费用（LECS，lifetime expected cost for survivors）。存活到特定年龄的人均余生期望医疗费用是由该队列在该年龄时的尚存者余生期望医疗费用除以该年龄时的尚存者队列样本量，则

在 x 岁时按出生时计算的某年龄尚存者人均余生期望医疗费用：$\text{LECS}_a = \sum\limits_{x=a}^{95}\left(\dfrac{C_x L_x}{l_a}\right)$；在 x 岁时某年龄尚存者人均余生期望医疗费用占尚存者人均终生期望医疗费用比值：$\text{RLECS}_a = \text{LECS}_a / \text{LECS}_0 = \sum\limits_{x=a}^{95}\left(\dfrac{C_x L_x}{l_a}\right) \bigg/ \sum\limits_{x=0}^{95}\left(\dfrac{C_x L_x}{l_0}\right)$。

二、终生医疗费用模型测算结果

（一）人口学及费用主要特征

2015 年上海市常住人口数为 2 415.27 万人。0～14 岁儿童少年组 217.28 万人，占总人口的 8.99%；15～59 岁中青年组 1 727.29 万人，占总人口的 71.52%；60 岁及以上老年人口组 470.70 万人，占总人口的 19.49%，其中 90 岁以上组人口最少，为 10.50 万人，占总人口的 0.43%（见图 4-1）。

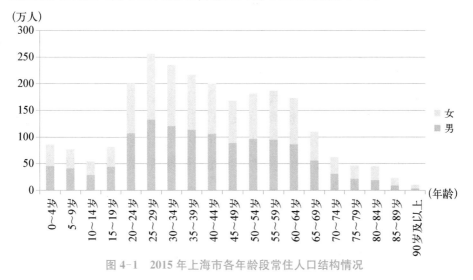

图 4-1　2015 年上海市各年龄段常住人口结构情况

与常住人口年龄构成比较,19.5%的老年人口发生的门急诊人次占总量的52.2%,出院人数占总量的45.3%,说明总体上老年人口消耗医疗资源较多。费用在各年龄段的分布规律与服务量趋同,但相对于服务量,集中度更高,19.5%的老年人口发生的门急诊费用占总量的63.2%,住院费用占总量的52.8%。医疗总费用构成与人口构成相比,50岁以下费用构成远低于人口构成,50~54岁组两者构成比相近,55岁及以上各组费用构成比均大于人口构成比(见图4-2)。

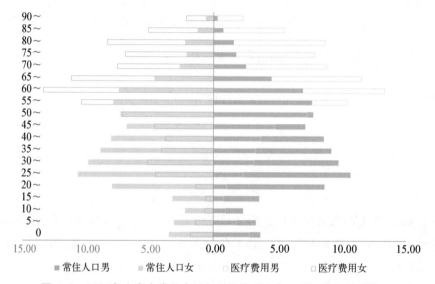

图4-2　2015年上海市常住人口与医疗费用在各年龄阶段的构成情况

(二) 常住人口终生医疗费用测算

1. 门急诊费用终生医疗费用测算

寿命表模拟的终生门急诊费用中,门急诊人均医疗费用、门急诊死亡人均医疗费用基本呈现随年龄逐渐增长的趋势,其中门急诊人均医疗费用的增长较为平缓,而门急诊死亡人均医疗费用略有波动。0岁组门急诊医疗费用为0,可能是由于婴幼儿死亡绝大多数发生在住院期间,在收集数据的2015年内,门急诊没有发生婴幼儿死亡。

由结果可知,人均余生期望门急诊医疗费用与尚存者人均余生期望门急诊医疗费用随着年龄增长不断降低,表明随着年龄增长,个人能够消耗的终生医疗费用不断减少,同一年龄组的后者略高于前者(见表4-1、图4-3)。

表 4-1 2015 年上海市门急诊费用与终生医疗费用模拟结果

年龄组（岁）	尚存人数（人）	死亡人数（人）	生存人年数（人年）	生存总人年数（人年）	门急诊人均医疗费用（元）	门急诊死亡人均医疗费用（元）	年龄别门急诊医疗费用（元）	人均余生期望门急诊医疗费用（元）	尚存者人均余生期望门急诊医疗费用（元）
0～	100 000	483	99 604	8 292 764	1 051.04	0.00	104 687 872.51	280 890.92	280 890.92
1～	99 517	185	397 699	8 193 160	1 051.04	2 149.12	417 998 004.71	279 844.04	281 198.26
5～	99 332	89	496 440	7 795 461	1 481.42	96.14	735 438 070.33	275 664.06	277 516.58
10～	99 243	98	495 974	7 299 021	906.75	149.10	449 723 163.77	268 309.68	270 354.84
15～	99 146	125	495 417	6 803 048	324.21	890.03	160 618 079.88	263 812.45	266 083.81
20～	99 021	100	494 854	6 307 630	198.22	1 005.72	98 092 075.71	262 206.27	264 797.81
25～	98 920	117	494 309	5 812 777	742.90	2 051.35	367 222 475.01	261 225.34	264 073.67
30～	98 803	158	493 621	5 318 468	1 128.07	1 775.84	556 837 142.60	257 553.12	260 670.28
35～	98 645	214	492 691	4 824 847	1 051.76	2 209.87	518 193 836.28	251 984.75	255 440.42
40～	98 431	340	491 303	4 332 156	1 024.48	2 787.41	503 331 728.56	246 802.81	250 727.50
45～	98 090	591	488 974	3 840 853	1 494.60	2 179.93	730 821 781.85	241 769.49	246 463.04
50～	97 499	1 003	484 989	3 351 879	2 335.46	1 958.56	113 267 2828.48	234 461.28	240 454.90
55～	96 496	1 741	478 128	2 866 890	3 535.33	2 709.59	169 0338 044.53	223 134.55	231 187.45
60～	94 755	2 468	467 605	2 388 762	5 118.67	2 554.31	2 393 518 261.30	206 231.17	217 580.51
65～	92 287	3 873	451 754	1 921 157	6 899.37	2 692.25	3 116 820 247.66	182 295.98	197 418.05
70～	88 414	6 623	425 515	1 469 403	8 648.06	2 695.91	3 679 877 290.27	151 127.78	170 729.28
75～	81 791	11 839	379 359	1 043 888	10 263.32	2 862.33	3 893 480 513.62	114 329.01	139 366.78
80～	69 952	17 472	306 079	664 530	11 663.56	3 187.17	3 569 973 398.82	75 394.20	106 983.85
85～	52 480	22 289	206 677	358 450	12 200.24	3 251.86	2 521 513 324.01	39 694.47	74 256.62
90～	30 191	30 191	151 773	151 773	9 540.14	3 006.17	1 447 933 596.92	14 479.34	47 958.76

注：生存人年数为该年龄组尚存人数的生存人年数，生存总人年数为从该年龄组到终生年龄组的生存人年数之和。

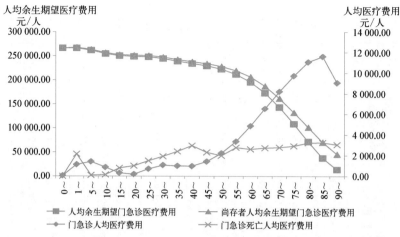

图 4-3   2015 年上海市常住人口人均医疗费用与余生期望医疗费用(门急诊)

　　60～64 岁组尚存者人均余生门急诊期望医疗费用占人均终生门急诊医疗
费用的比值为 77.46%,表明 60～64 岁组中,每人从现在到其死亡的期望门急
诊医疗费用占其一辈子门急诊医疗费用的 77.46%,即约有高达八成的门急诊
医疗费用被用于 60～64 岁以后的老年期(见图 4-4)。

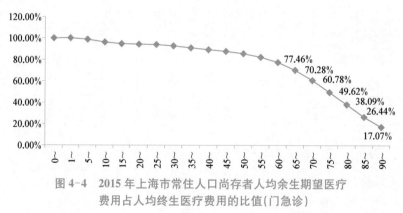

图 4-4   2015 年上海市常住人口尚存者人均余生期望医疗
费用占人均终生医疗费用的比值(门急诊)

2. 住院费用

　　与门急诊比较发现,住院死亡人均医疗费用较高,不仅远远高于门急诊死
亡人均医疗费用,还高于住院人均医疗费用。最高峰出现在 1～4 岁组,高达
156 299.8 元/人。和门急诊不同的是,虽然住院人均医疗费用也呈逐渐上升
的趋势,但住院死亡人均医疗费用下降趋势明显,较大值均出现在 50～54 岁
组前,这可能是由于为更尽力地挽救儿童、青年、中年人群的生命,对其临终前
投入的医疗资源相对老年人群更大(见表 4-2、图 4-5)。

表 4-2 住院费用寿命表结果

年龄组（岁）	尚存人数（人）	死亡人数（人）	生存人年数（人年）	生存总人年数（人年）	住院人均医疗费用（元）	住院死亡人均医疗费用（元）	年龄别住院医疗费用（元）	人均余生期望住院医疗费用（元）	尚存者人均余生期望住院医疗费用（元）
0～	100 000	483	99 604	8 292 764	1 695.98	21 795.98	168 926 425.91	202 899.25	202 793.98
1～	99 517	185	397 699	8 193 160	1 695.98	156 299.80	674 489 864.74	201 209.99	201 896.67
5～	99 332	89	496 440	7 795 461	660.95	104 970.70	328 123 411.76	194 465.09	195 677.99
10～	99 243	98	495 974	7 299 021	613.74	102 142.90	304 401 270.27	191 183.86	192 540.88
15～	99 146	125	495 417	6 803 048	520.64	91 988.93	257 934 970.85	188 139.85	189 644.49
20～	99 021	100	494 854	6 307 630	429.50	89 360.27	212 539 587.32	185 560.50	187 304.57
25～	98 920	117	494 309	5 812 777	676.94	129 178.30	334 619 194.87	183 435.10	185 283.65
30～	98 803	158	493 621	5 318 468	731.96	82 347.93	361 308 948.01	180 088.91	182 139.00
35～	98 645	214	492 691	4 824 847	722.11	100 367.90	355 779 105.12	176 475.82	178 681.17
40～	98 431	340	491 303	4 332 156	914.72	69 192.16	449 404 617.92	172 918.03	175 435.20
45～	98 090	591	488 974	3 840 853	1 435.38	70 897.88	701 862 692.02	168 423.98	171 275.50
50～	97 499	1 003	484 989	3 351 879	1 801.75	69 515.20	873 829 639.38	161 405.35	164 830.24
55～	96 496	1 741	478 128	2 866 890	2 265.67	73 046.32	1 083 278 665.02	152 667.06	156 892.00
60～	94 755	2 468	467 605	2 388 762	2 901.23	68 650.87	1 356 631 090.64	141 834.27	147 897.66
65～	92 287	3 873	451 754	1 921 157	3 849.65	66 740.11	1 739 097 068.14	128 267.96	136 186.94
70～	88 414	6 623	425 515	1 469 403	4 985.53	61 833.32	2 121 414 065.72	110 876.99	120 774.27
75～	81 791	11 839	379 359	1 043 888	6 294.61	55 453.36	2 387 916 135.31	89 662.85	101 596.75
80～	69 952	17 472	306 079	664 530	7 853.98	51 858.80	2 403 941 629.06	65 783.69	81 088.16
85～	52 480	22 289	206 677	358 450	11 021.96	54 490.73	2 277 989 937.42	41 744.27	56 401.00
90～	30 191	30 191	151 773	151 773	12 495.24	55 272.54	1 896 437 162.48	18 964.37	62 814.19

注：生存人年数为该年龄组尚存人数的生存人年数；生存总人年数为从该年龄组到终生的生存人年数之和。

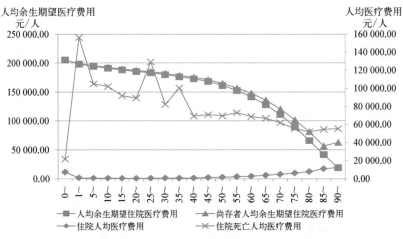

图 4-5　2015 年上海市常住人口人均医疗费用与余生期望医疗费用(住院)

尚存者人均余生期望住院医疗费用占人均终生住院医疗费用的比值，60～64 岁组达 72.93%，较门急诊低 4.53 个百分点，说明 60～64 岁组的老人从现在到其死亡的期望门急诊医疗费用占其一辈子门急诊医疗费用的 72.93%。75 岁及以上组的四个年龄组，从现在到死亡，其所花费的住院医疗费用占其一辈子医疗费用的比重均略高于门急诊比重(见图 4-6)。

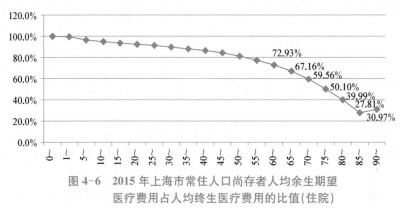

图 4-6　2015 年上海市常住人口尚存者人均余生期望
医疗费用占人均终生医疗费用的比值(住院)

3. 总医疗费用

将门急诊、住院合并来看，人均总医疗费用随着年龄的增长缓慢增加。但是由于住院费用远高于门急诊，死亡人均总医疗费用受住院死亡人均医疗费用的影响较大，呈现出与其类似的波动特征，同时也远远高于人均总医疗费用。剔除死亡人数与医疗费用后，除 0～1 岁组外，同一年龄组尚存者人均余生期望总医疗费用均略高于人均余生期望门急诊医疗费用(见表 4-3、图 4-7)。

表4-3　总医疗费用寿命表结果

年龄组（岁）	尚存人数（人）	死亡人数（人）	生存人年数（人年）	生存总人年数（人年）	人均总医疗费用（元）	死亡人均总医疗费用（元）	年龄别总医疗费用（元）	人均余生期望总医疗费用（元）	尚存者人均余生期望总医疗费用（元）
0～	100 000	483	99 604	8 292 764	2 747.02	21 795.98	273 614 298.42	483 790.17	483 684.90
1～	99 517	185	397 699	8 193 160	2 747.02	158 448.92	1 092 487 869.45	481 054.03	483 094.93
5～	99 332	89	496 440	7 795 461	2 142.38	105 066.84	1 063 561 482.09	470 129.15	473 194.57
10～	99 243	98	495 974	7 299 021	1 520.49	102 292.00	754 124 434.04	459 493.54	462 895.72
15～	99 146	125	495 417	6 803 048	844.85	92 878.96	418 553 050.74	451 952.29	455 728.30
20～	99 021	100	494 854	6 307 630	627.72	90 365.99	310 631 663.03	447 766.76	452 102.37
25～	98 920	117	494 309	5 812 777	1 419.84	131 229.65	701 841 669.88	444 660.44	449 357.33
30～	98 803	158	493 621	5 318 468	1 860.02	84 123.77	918 146 090.61	437 642.03	442 809.28
35～	98 645	214	492 691	4 824 847	1 773.88	102 577.77	873 972 941.40	428 460.57	434 121.59
40～	98 431	340	491 303	4 332 156	1 939.20	71 979.57	952 736 346.47	419 720.84	426 162.69
45～	98 090	591	488 974	3 840 853	2 929.98	73 077.81	1 432 684 473.87	410 193.47	417 738.54
50～	97 499	1 003	484 989	3 351 879	4 137.21	71 473.76	2 006 502 467.86	395 866.63	405 285.14
55～	96 496	1 741	478 128	2 866 890	5 800.99	75 755.91	2 773 616 709.56	375 801.60	388 079.45
60～	94 755	2 468	467 605	2 388 762	8 019.90	71 205.18	3 750 149 351.94	348 065.44	365 478.17
65～	92 287	3 873	451 754	1 921 157	10 749.03	69 432.36	4 855 917 315.80	310 563.94	333 604.99
70～	88 414	6 623	425 515	1 469 403	13 633.59	64 529.23	5 801 291 355.99	262 004.77	291 503.55
75～	81 791	11 839	379 359	1 043 888	16 557.94	58 315.69	6 281 396 648.93	203 991.86	240 963.53
80～	69 952	17 472	306 079	664 530	19 517.54	55 045.97	5 973 915 027.88	141 177.89	188 072.01
85～	52 480	22 289	206 677	358 450	23 222.20	57 742.59	4 799 503 261.42	81 438.74	130 657.61
90～	30 191	30 191	151 773	151 773	22 035.38	58 278.71	3 344 370 759.41	33 443.71	110 772.95

注：生存人年数为该年龄组尚存人数的生存人年数；生存总人年数为从该年龄组到终生的生存人年数之和。

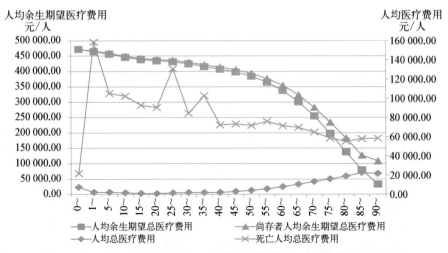

图 4-7　2015 年上海市常住人口人均医疗费用与余生期望医疗费用(总)

60～64 岁组、80～84 岁组的尚存者人均余生期望总医疗费用占人均终生总医疗费用比值分别为 75.56%、38.88%。90 岁以上组尚存者人均余生期望总医疗费用占人均终生总医疗费用比值也达 22.90%，说明活到 90 岁以上的老人，直到死亡，其所花费的医疗费用仍约占其终生医疗费用的二成(见图 4-8)。

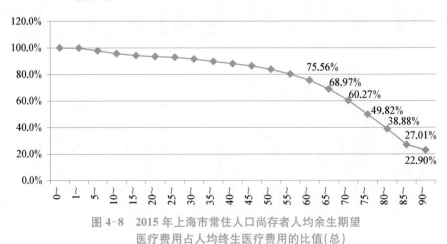

图 4-8　2015 年上海市常住人口尚存者人均余生期望
医疗费用占人均终生医疗费用的比值(总)

三、启示与借鉴

(一)国际比较显示,上海市老年人群的医疗费用在终生费用中的比例较高

研究结果初步显示,就终生医疗费用来看,花费在老年期的医疗费用(不

论门急诊、住院及总体)占其一生所花费医疗费用的大部分(八成左右),这表明终生医疗费用在老龄阶段趋于集中,也从一个侧面反映出老龄人口使用了较大比例的社会医疗资源。在对发达国家的比较分析中,我们发现,虽然发达国家老龄人口相较于其他人群的医疗费用集中趋势也基本明晰,但差异程度较上海缓和。

终生医疗费用模型基于横断面数据测算,医疗服务价格、医疗技术进步等重要影响因素没有纳入模型,其模拟所得的终生医疗费用只能反映当前的费用水平,但老年人余生期望医疗费用相对比值与其他地区比较,可以反映当前医疗资源在不同年龄段配置的合理性。

例如,Alemayehu 等(2004)对美国密歇根州的研究显示,该地区 65 岁以上人口医疗费用占终生医疗费用的 1/2。上海地区的费用分析显示,60～64 岁组尚存者人均余生门急诊期望医疗费用占人均终生门急诊医疗费用的比值为 77.46%;60～64 岁组尚存者人均余生期望住院医疗费用占人均终生住院医疗费用的比值达 72.93%。排除年份和方法学因素的混杂,可以看出,上海地区老年人群的医疗费用在终生费用中的比例远高于美国密歇根州相应比例。

(二) 80 岁及以上老年人群医疗费用预期主要流向住院,而 80 岁以下老年人群医疗费用预期主要流向门诊

由结果可知,80～84 岁组从其现在到死亡花费的医疗费用占到了终生费用的 38.88%,其中门急诊为 38.09%,住院为 39.99%,略高于门诊。自 75 岁及以上组起,四个高龄年龄组均为住院人均余生期望总医疗费用占人均终生医疗总费用的比值高于门急诊,而其余老年组呈现出相反的特征。这说明,高龄老年人群的人均余生期望医疗费用主要发生在住院,而相对低龄的老年人群(60～74 岁)的人均余生期望医疗费用主要发生在门诊,这一结果也较为符合本市老年人群医疗服务利用的实际情况。

(三) 推进就医、养老进一步下沉社区,充分调动利用社区资源

老年人群在不同机构间的诊疗缺乏连贯性,导致出现医疗资源浪费,这是部分导致医疗费用在老年人口中持续走高的原因之一。尽管上海市大力推行"1+1+1"(一家社区医院＋一家二级医院＋一家三级医院)的就医模式和分级诊疗制度,但收效并不明显。社区是构建适宜的养老服务体系的重要基石,为使养老服务下沉社区,2016 年上海市老龄工作委员会办公室和上海市民政

局联合颁布《关于加强社区综合为老服务中心建设的指导意见》（沪老龄办发〔2016〕5 号）。其中提出，鼓励社区综合为老服务中心与周边医院、社区卫生服务中心、康复护理等机构合作，引入社区卫生服务站（点、室）、护理站、其他康复服务，或与已有的医疗服务机构综合设置，加强在社区层面的医养结合。

举例来说，上海市虹口区曲阳社区在长期实践中摸索出了一套可供借鉴的模式。该社区打造"一站式"综合为老服务平台，集合了传统的窗口咨询、文化娱乐等服务，同时引入了养老服务综合评估、社区家庭医生制、家庭养老介入服务等新功能。除提供居家康复、家庭病床、临终关怀等上门服务外，更具备日间照料中心，依托专业康复护理组织，提供护理、康复运动等服务，并为中度以上的社区失能失智老人提供包括助餐、助洁、医疗介护等在内的社会化上门安养服务。建议继续探索以健康结果为导向的整合型医疗服务模式，充分利用社区资源，推进分级诊疗建设。

（四）推动长期护理保险制度，促进老年照护公共服务供给

自 2017 年 1 月起，上海市长期护理保险制度在徐汇、普陀、金山三区启动试点，2018 年起推广至全市。这不仅给养老公共服务盘子增加了资源，还对既有的养老服务资源进行系统集成，将本市的机构、社区、居家养老服务资源，整合至同一个调度和结算系统里[①]。长期护理保险将作为独立的第六大保险，与养老保险、医疗保险、失业保险、工伤保险、生育保险共同构架起上海市社会保险体系。

推进长期护理保险需要秉持顶层设计，坚持循序渐进的路径，规避制度设计"碎片化"，保证长期护理保险项目与养老保险、医疗保险等项目的协调统一。对于普通人群，需要根据其对护理服务的需求程度，分级别进行支付与补偿；对于特殊人群，如失独老人、低保低收入老人等，应予以优先保障与满足。坚持"小步走、快步走"，分类别、分阶段、有重点地逐步推进制度建设。同时在国家政策框架下，结合上海实际，支持和鼓励商业保险公司大力开发商业性长期护理保险产品，促进老年照护服务供给。

（五）控制住院费用，引导优化医疗费用使用结构

与国际先进国家的比较显示，上海市老年医疗费用存在节约的空间，特别

---

① World Health Organization. 关于老龄化与健康的全球报告. 2015.

是高龄老年人群医疗费用重点是控制住院费用。国际经验发现,护理及康复对住院服务有很大的补充替代作用,更对老龄患者的精神心理护理带来远期裨益。

事实上,上海市目前已经具备了一套针对老年人口的医疗服务提供体系框架。医院、基层医疗卫生机构、公共卫生机构和其他机构,为满足老年人的预防、医疗、护理和康复需求等提供相应服务。此外,还大力推动建立安宁疗护(临终关怀)项目,设立机构和居家舒缓疗护床位,为老年人在生命末期提供临终关怀。然而,尽管框架体系已经存在,但资源整合尚待发展,护理及康复服务的利用尚有待提高,亟待相关部门整合医疗服务资源、优化为老养老服务结构。建议有关部门积极深化推广相关先进经验,加大住院医疗服务的替代服务的发展。

第 五 章

临终医疗行为及费用一瞥

【导读】

　　死亡是伴随每个人生命历程的巨大阴影,是任何人都无法回避的最终归宿。随着现代医学的发展,越来越多的死亡发生在医疗机构里。然而,发展中国家鲜有人对临终前人们的就医行为开展系统性研究。本章聚焦上海市临终前 1 年的患者,探讨不同年龄、性别患者间住院服务和费用的差异,及住院费用随距离死亡时间的变化情况。结果显示,2015 年,上海市各医疗机构内死亡的患者共有 43 765 人,占 2015 年上海市总死亡人口的 35%。总的来说,较年轻的死亡者住院费用高于年龄较大的死亡者,死亡人群与全人群的住院费用比从 44 岁以下人群的 120 倍降至 85 岁及以上人群的 5 倍。在三级医疗机构中,全人群的人均住院费用与年龄成正比,而终末期患者的人均住院费用则随年龄上升而下降;在二级医疗机构中,2 个人群的年龄分布则均随年龄的上升而上升。在不同死因组患者中,死于脑卒中和心肌梗死的患者费用较低,死于癌症的患者费用高于其他患者。临终前 1 年的住院费用中超过 40% 发生在死亡前 1 个月内。由于临终费用的年龄别、疾病别、费用结构差异的特点,接近死亡效应与老龄化的综合作用也会呈现不同的结果。可以肯定的是,这两种效应的叠加效果给老龄化背景下的医疗费用预测带来了更大的挑战。

中国社会的老龄化步伐正在加快。全国 60 岁及以上人口占比从 2000 年的
7.0% 上升到 2015 年的 16.1%[1]。2015 年人口抽样调查结果显示,上海市常住人
口中,60 岁及以上老年人占 19.5%,65 岁及以上占 12.3%。人口结构的变化导
致临终前医疗需求的增加。然而到目前为止,发展中国家鲜有关于终末期医疗
费用的研究。国际研究显示医疗费用具有"接近死亡效应"(Proximity to Death,
PTD)。临终前患者会使用较多的医疗卫生资源,导致临终前医疗费用高于生存
者的医疗费用[2][3][4][5]。Zweifel 等提出[6],老年人发生死亡的概率大,临终前医
疗费用突增使老年组的人均医疗费用高于年轻组,接近死亡效应这个不相干事
实造成老龄化推高医疗费用的假象。根据现有研究,接近死亡效应具有距离死
亡时间差异、年龄别、疾病别、费用结构和地区差异等特点[7][8][9][10]。深入了解终

① 国家卫生和计划生育委员会.中国卫生和计划生育统计年鉴 2016[M].北京:中国
协和医科大学出版社,2016: 336.
② McGrail K, Bo Green, Barer M L, et al. Age, costs of acute and long-term care
and proximity to death: evidence for 1987—1988 and 1994—1995 in British Columbia[J].
Age and Ageing, 2000,29(3): 249—253.
③ Barnato A E, McClellan M B, Garber C, et al. Trends in inpatient treatment
intensity among medicare beneficiaries at the end of life[J]. Health Services Research,
2004, 39(2): 363—376.
④ Polder J J, Barendregt J J, van Oers H, Health care costs in the last year of life-
The Dutch experience[J]. Social Science & Medicine, 2006, 63(7): 1720—1731.
⑤ Blakely T, Atkinson J, Kvizhinadze G, et al. Health system costs by sex, age and
proximity to death, and implications for estimation of future expenditure [J]. New
Zealand Medical Journal, 2014, 127(1393): 12—25.
⑥ Zweifel P, Felder S, Meiers M. Ageing of population and health care
expenditure: A red herring? [J]. Health Economics, 1999, 8(6): 485—496.
⑦ Shugarman L R, Campbell D E, Bird C E, et al. Differences in medicare expenditures
during the last 3 years of life[J].Journal of General Internal Medicine, 2004, 19(2): 127—135.
⑧ Gozalo P, Plotzke M, Mor V. Changes in medicare costs with the growthof
hospice care in nursing homes [J]. New England Journal of Medicine,2015, 372(19):
1823—1831.
⑨ Spillman B C, Lubitz J. The effect of longevity on spending for acute and long-
term care[J]. New England Journal of Medicine, 2000, 342(19): 1409—1415.
⑩ Wong A, van Baal P H M, Boshuizen H C. et al. Exploring the influence of
proximity to death on disease-specific hospital expenditures: A carpaccio of red herrings
[J]. Health Economics, 2011, 20(4): 379—400.

末期医疗费用特征，以及人口老龄化和接近死亡效应的交互作用对医疗费用产生的影响，将有助于更好的政策应对。上海是全国最早进入老龄化的地区之一，在卫生管理和医疗体系改革方面积累了大量经验。鉴于现有的研究都是在发达国家开展的，本章旨在利用上海市个人层面的医疗大数据，比较终末期患者及全人群住院费用的差异，描述不同性别、不同死因患者费用的年龄分布，并研究终末期费用的接近死亡效应。

一、临终期医疗行为追踪方法

上海市卫生和计划生育委员会信息中心健康信息网数据平台汇集了上海市所有医疗机构的患者就诊记录，包括各级各类医院、社区卫生服务机构、妇幼保健院（所）和专科疾病防治院（所、站）等。我们利用该数据平台追踪 2015 年 1 月 1 日至 2015 年 12 月 31 日在医疗机构内死亡人群临终前 1 年的住院服务利用情况，并分析其费用特点。本章中所指的终末期住院费用就是死亡人群临终前 1 年所产生的住院费用，死亡人群最后一次住院记录的主要诊断作为其死因。同时，以 5 岁为组距收集 2015 年全市常住人口全年龄段住院服务利用和住院费用信息，并与死亡人口临终前 1 年的住院服务利用和费用情况进行比较。常住人口总数来源于上海市统计年鉴，常住人口结构数据来源于上海市统计局 2015 年常住人口抽样调查数据。

我们计算了死亡人群不同性别、年龄、死因组的住院费用，以及死亡前 12 个月的住院费用分布，在与全人群住院费用进行比较时，仅计算了 2015 年产生的费用。对于全人群，我们计算了 2015 年上海市常住人口不同性别、年龄组的住院费用，这其中可能有部分人口在 2015 年死于医疗机构以外的地方，没有纳入死亡人群范畴，可能会缩小终末期费用与全人群费用的差异。使用 T 检验对连续性资料进行统计检验，卡方检验用于计数资料，皮尔逊相关系数（r）进行相关性检验，描述性和统计分析均使用 STATA 13.0 完成，设置显著性水平 α 为 0.05。

二、临终期人群的就诊行为及费用结构

（一）死亡人群基本特征

2015 年在上海市各医疗机构内死亡的患者共有 43 765 人，占 2015 年上海市总死亡人口的 35%。表 5-1 列出了这部分死亡人群的基本特征，其中 65

岁及以上老年人占比达到 81.77%，男性占比为 55.56%。在终末期患者的死因构成方面，死于癌症、循环系统和呼吸系统疾病的患者人数最多。参保类型的构成方面，81.80% 参加了城镇职工医保，10.99% 参加了城镇居民医保，2.62% 参加了新农合，与全人群的参保类型构成基本一致。

表 5-1　2015 年上海市各医疗机构内死亡人群基本特征

	人　数	占比（%）
死亡年龄		
0～44	657	1.50
45～64	7 324	16.73
65～74	6 497	14.85
75～84	14 425	32.96
85 及以上	14 862	33.96
性别		
男	24 312	55.56
女	19 453	44.44
参保类型		
城镇职工基本医疗保险	35 800	81.80
城镇居民基本医疗保险	4 811	10.99
新型农村合作医疗	1 145	2.62
其他	2 009	4.59
死亡原因		
癌症	15 115	34.54
循环系统疾病	11 464	26.19
呼吸系统疾病	9 825	22.45
其他	7 361	16.82

（二）年龄、性别与机构分布

表 5-2 列出了 2015 年上海市终末期患者全人群与死亡人群不同性别、年龄组的人均住院费用。在全人群中，不同年龄组的人均住院费用差异较大，从 5～9 岁组的 660.90 元到 90 岁组的 12 506.01 元，相差达到 18 倍。临终前 1 年，

女性所花费的住院费用低于男性（$T=-15.1244$，$P<0.05$）。

表 5-2 2015 年上海市终末期患者和全人群人均住院费用（单位：元）

年龄组	终末期患者			全 人 群		
	女性	男性	合计	女性	男性	合计
0~1	19 623.37	**23 968.59**	21 795.98	6 297.47	**8 326.82**	7 346.23
1~4	89 874.71	**189 512.40**	156 299.80	802.48	**1 063.99**	941.50
5~9	20 694.48	**189 247.00**	104 970.70	557.47	**751.31**	660.90
10~14	59 991.98	**144 293.90**	102 142.90	490.77	**723.90**	614.36
15~19	72 963.52	**109 284.80**	91 988.93	483.55	**551.90**	520.68
20~24	**132 130.60**	46 589.95	89 360.27	**525.51**	346.93	429.63
25~29	114 480.20	**145 772.90**	129 178.30	**918.66**	451.80	677.44
30~34	71 834.37	**94 088.08**	82 347.93	**953.00**	522.47	731.69
35~39	100 028.40	**101 588.50**	100 804.00	**833.49**	622.54	722.74
40~44	**72 410.62**	67 288.27	69 192.16	**960.94**	874.39	914.87
45~49	69 475.48	**71 753.41**	70 897.88	**1 448.27**	1 416.07	1 431.25
50~54	67 889.58	**70 312.47**	69 515.20	1 753.49	**1 853.37**	1 806.45
55~59	**78 784.55**	70 377.30	73 046.32	2 007.69	**2 510.41**	2 263.87
60~64	**69 010.31**	68 579.38	68 714.02	2 477.76	**3 325.38**	2 900.72
65~69	65 363.48	**67 529.48**	66 833.64	3 298.64	**4 365.77**	3 842.79
70~74	61 177.23	**62 269.84**	61 881.54	4 211.34	**5 761.96**	4 987.65
75~79	53 742.18	**56 846.89**	55 537.20	5 537.68	**7 117.16**	6 278.90
80~84	48 796.38	**54 885.68**	52 024.21	7 049.34	**8 984.74**	7 876.59
85~89	46 198.93	**64 527.71**	54 927.92	9 144.40	**14 047.89**	11 030.83
≥90	39 589.67	**73 613.80**	54 164.27	9 399.12	**18 827.54**	12 506.01

注：加粗的数值表示每一年龄组两个性别组中费用较高的值。

20%的死亡人群临终前 1 年的住院费用超过 16 万元，累计费用占死亡人群临终前 1 年总住院费用的 56.5%。住院费用前 1%的终末期患者（约 438 人）累计住院费用达 3.26 亿元，约合人均 74.39 万元，住院费用前 5%的终末期患者（约 2 189 人）累计住院费用达到 8.64 亿元，约合人均 39.49 万元。

　　研究发现,终末期住院费用与患者的死亡年龄成反比(见图5-1),44岁以下人群临终前1年住院费用为人均8.86万元,90岁以上组则降为人均5.42万元($r=-0.0894$,$P<0.05$)。这一反比关系在女性患者中更为明显($r=-0.1746$,$P<0.05$),男性患者超过85岁以后,其人均住院费用有所回升,这其中的差异部分是由于临终前男性和女性对医疗机构级别的选择所导致的。总体上来说,除了55～64岁组,男性的终末期住院费用高于女性。

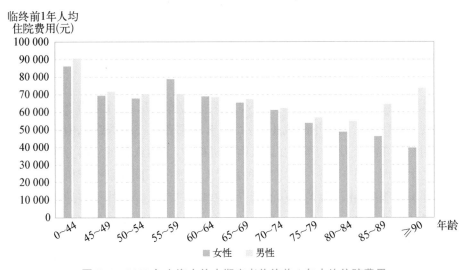

图5-1　2015年上海市终末期患者临终前1年人均住院费用

　　死亡人群与全人群的住院费用比值与年龄高度相关,图5-2显示该比值随年龄上升逐渐下降,从120多倍(44岁以下)到5倍(85岁及以上)。在50～79岁的女性人群中,死亡者与全人群的费用比值高于男性,主要是由于女性整体的医疗费用较低,而非女性临终前耗费了更多的医疗资源。

　　终末期患者在不同机构的住院费用呈现出不同的年龄分布特点。在三级医疗机构,终末期患者的住院费用随年龄上升而逐渐下降($r=-0.0678$,$P<0.05$),二级医疗机构的人均住院费用则随年龄的上升而提高($r=0.0128$,$P<0.05$)。79岁以后,二级医疗机构的人均住院费用甚至超过了三级医疗机构。而在全人群中,总体住院费用随年龄上升而上升,79岁以后,二级医疗机构的人均住院费用超过三级医疗机构。

　　终末期患者与全人群在不同机构的住院费用呈现出不同的年龄分布(见

费用比值

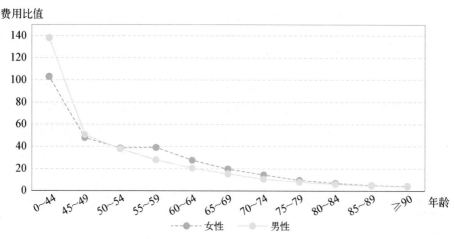

图 5-2　2015 年死亡人群与全人群人均住院费用比值

图 5-3）。在三级医疗机构中，两组人群的年龄分布相反，即全人群在三级医疗机构的人均住院费用与年龄成正比，而终末期患者在三级医疗机构的人均住院费用则随年龄上升而下降；在二级医疗机构中，两组人群的年龄分布则均随年龄的上升而上升。这种差异在某种程度上反映了不同级别医疗机构所提供的不同类型服务，由于收治疾病类型存在差异，三级医疗机构更多地提供高技术含量的医疗服务，而二级医疗机构则更多地提供康复、护理等资源消耗程度较低的服务。

人均住院费用(元)

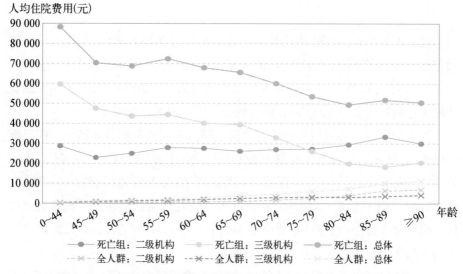

图 5-3　2015 年不同级别医疗机构全人群与死亡组患者人均住院费用

　　总体上来说,终末期患者在三级医疗机构住院的次数随年龄的上升而下降(见图 5-4、图 5-5)。然而 85 岁及以上男性在三级医疗机构住院次数的占比却开始升高,从 85～89 岁组的 18.77% 上升到 90 岁以上组的 26.28%(见图 5-5)。鉴于三级医疗机构的人均住院费用要高于低级别医疗机构(见表 5-3),临终前对于医疗机构选择的差异可能导致不同性别人群间的费用差异。

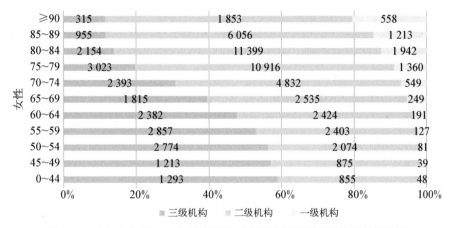

图 5-4　2015 年上海市女性终末期患者在不同级别医疗机构的住院次数

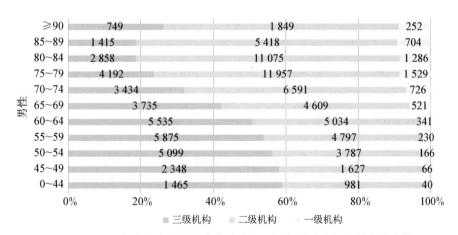

图 5-5　2015 年上海市男性终末期患者在不同级别医疗机构的住院次数

表 5-3　2015 年上海市终末期患者在不同级别医疗机构的人均住院费用

医疗机构级别	患者人数	比例(%)	人均住院费用(元)
三级	16 439	28.49	85 668.86($P<0.05$)
二级	35 192	60.98	63 397.06($P<0.05$)
一级	6 080	10.54	24 970.29

(三) 性别与死因组

我们通过死亡人群最后一次住院的主诊断来确定其死因,通过 ICD-10 编码的前三位确定疾病类别。表 5-4 列出了死亡人群的前 14 位死因,死于这 14 种疾病的患者占死亡人群的 61.77%。死于脑卒中和心肌梗死的患者费用较低,主要是由于这 2 种疾病致死率较高。14 个死因组患者的人均费用差异显著($F=19.47$,$P<0.05$),提示我们,不同死因组间患者费用的变异度大于某个特定组别内的变异度。

表 5-4　2015 年不同死因组患者人均住院费用

类　　别	人均费用(元)			总　费　用	
	女性	男性	合计	金额(亿元)	占比(%)
直肠癌	81 758	89 820	87 032	0.56	1.69
结肠癌	80 197	90 790	85 918	1.03	3.11
胃癌	78 384	86 764	83 572	1.41	4.26
呼吸衰竭	73 415	86 115	80 560	0.85	2.57
慢性阻塞性肺病	67 397	85 682	79 631	1.98	6.01
脑血管病后遗症	75 308	83 286	79 048	0.84	2.54
其他呼吸系统疾病	65 008	89 409	77 853	2.54	7.68
胰腺癌	72 942	80 654	77 130	0.86	2.60
慢性缺血性心脏病	65 251	91 181	76 452	2.51	7.59
肺癌	68 576	77 923	75 313	2.76	8.35
肺炎	57 341	85 144	72 717	1.45	4.38
肝癌	58 223	67 521	64 992	0.90	2.71
脑卒中	49 715	56 676	53 330	1.90	5.77

续　表

类　　别	人均费用(元)			总　费　用	
	女性	男性	合计	金额(亿元)	占比(%)
心肌梗死	47 126	54 445	51 262	0.34	1.04
其他	70 212	85 842	78 379	13.11	39.70
合计	67 124	82 099	75 443	33.02	100.00

不同死因组患者的住院费用同样随年龄的上升而下降,这一下降趋势在女性患者中更为明显,尤其是在 70 岁以后(见图 5-6)。而在男性患者中,不同死因组的患者住院费用在 84 岁以后均有所回升(见图 5-7)。癌症患者的住院费用随年龄下降的趋势更为明显,而死于循环系统疾病的患者住院费用较低,且各个年龄段患者的人均费用差异不大。

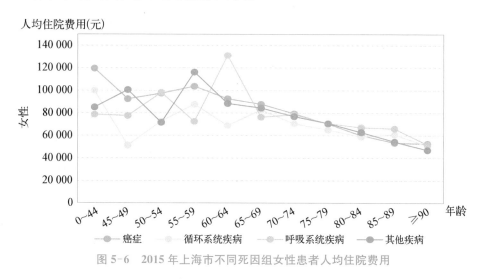

图 5-6　2015 年上海市不同死因组女性患者人均住院费用

在上海的医疗机构内,最常见的死因是癌症,占死亡人群的 34.54%。死于癌症的患者终末期住院费用高于其他死因组患者($F=50.42$,$P<0.05$)。

表 5-5　2015 年上海市不同死因组患者人均住院费用

性别	人均住院费用(元)			
	癌症	循环系统疾病	呼吸系统疾病	其他疾病
女性	77 232.13	60 074.92	64 942.88	64 565.17
男性	85 002.16	73 656.17	86 655.45	80 722.00

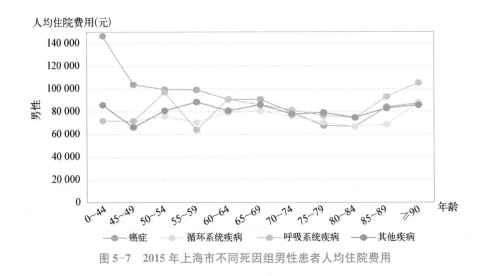

图 5-7　2015 年上海市不同死因组男性患者人均住院费用

（四）距离死亡时间

终末期患者临终前 1 年的住院费用中有 43% 发生在死亡前 1 个月，并且距离死亡时间越远，该占比越低。相应的，临终前患者的日均住院费用从死亡前 12 个月的 769 元增长到临终前 1 个月的 1 048 元，涨幅达到 26.6%（见图 5-8）。

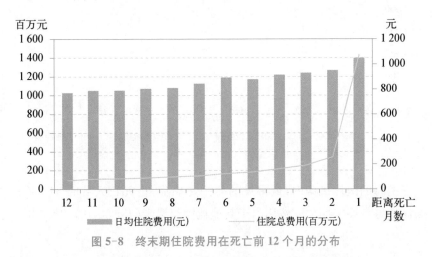

图 5-8　终末期住院费用在死亡前 12 个月的分布

图 5-9 显示了不同研究中 65 岁及以上老年人的终末期住院费用在临终前 4 个季度的分布情况。美国一项研究则显示[①]，患者临终前 1 年，约 60% 的

---

① Lubitz J D，Rily G F. Trends in Medicare payments in the last year of life[J]. New England Journal of Medicine，1993，328(15)：1092—1097.

医疗费用发生在临终前一个季度,这一比例自 1976 年开始就保持稳定。根据瑞士一项对老年人终末期费用的研究[①],65 岁及以上老年人临终前一年的医疗费用有 42%～49% 发生在临终前一个季度,20%～22% 发生在临终前第二季度,17%～19% 发生在临终前第三季度。我们的研究显示,65 岁及以上人群临终前 1 年的费用有 64% 发生在临终前一个季度,16% 发生在临终前第二季度,11% 发生在临终前第三季度,9% 发生在临终前第四季度,这一比例构成与美国的情况类似。与瑞士相比,上海市终末期医疗费用的接近死亡效应更为显著,即更高比例的医疗费用发生在更接近死亡的时间段内(见图 5-9)。由于瑞士政府对机构内医疗服务的补贴程度较高,随着死亡的临近,发生机构住院的概率提高,一定程度上缓解了医疗成本的急剧上升。

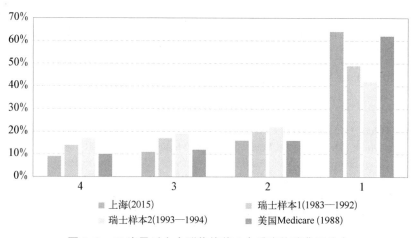

图 5-9　65 岁及以上人群临终前 4 个季度住院费用分布

三、临终期费用主要特点

(一) 较年轻者死亡成本更高

根据上海市 2015 年的数据分析结果,终末期患者临终前 1 年的住院费用随年龄的上升而下降,而这一下降幅度比其他研究结论所显示的幅度小,一方面由于上海的医疗机构床位以治疗性床位为主,护理、安宁疗护等床位设置较

---

① Zweifel P, Felder S, Meiers M. Ageing of population and health care expenditure: A red herring? [J]. Health Economics, 1999, 8(6): 485—496.

少，另一方面可能与中国文化中的孝道传统有关。在上海，95 岁以上的患者临终前 1 年的住院花费约为 65～70 岁组的 80%；根据 Polder[①] 和 Serup-Hansen[②] 对荷兰和丹麦相关情况的研究，这一占比更低。在德国，这一比例在 43%～47%左右[③]，而美国则在 40%[④]和 52%[⑤]左右。

　　死亡人群与全人群 2015 年的人均住院费用比值为平均 32.9 倍（4.3 到 119.5 倍），该值高于其他国家的研究结果。例如 Polder 发现死亡者与生存者医疗费用的平均比值为 13.5（5 到 30），而在丹麦的男性和女性群体中，该比值分别为 9.4 和 13.3。当我们缩小死亡人群的年龄范围，仅观察 65 岁及以上的老年人时，终末期患者与全市常住人口的住院费用比值为 4.3 到 17.4 倍，该结论与加拿大的一项研究结果比较相近，在加拿大，该比值为 2.5 到 16.6 倍[⑥]。

　　长久以来，经济学家就把健康视为人力资本的重要组成部分[⑦][⑧][⑨]。人力资本论的奠基者和创始人西奥多·W.舒尔茨认为，投资于健康来改善人力资本存量的质量，是促进经济增长的主要动力[⑩]。结合健康与医疗卫生服务需求理论，Grossman 认为健康是一种投资品，健康资本的增加可以使人们拥有更

---

①　Polder J J，Barendregt J J，van Oers H，Health care costs in the last year of life—The Dutch experience[J]. Social Science & Medicine，2006，63(7)：1720—1731.

②　Serup-Hansen N，Wickstrom J，Kristiansen I S. Future health care costs—Do health care costs during the last year of life matter？[J]. Health Policy，2002，62(2)：161—172.

③　Brockmann H. Why is less money spent on health care for the elderly than for the rest of the population？ Health care rationing in German hospitals[J]. Social Science and Medicine，2002，55(4)：593—608.

④　Riley G，Lubitz J，Prihoda R，et al. The use and costs of Medicare services by cause of death[J]. Inquiry，1987，24(3)：233—244.

⑤　Perls T T. Acute care costs of the oldest old[J]. Hospital Practice，1997，32(7)：123—137.

⑥　McGrail K，Green B，Barer M L，et al. Age，costs of acute and long-term care and proximity to death：evidence for 1987—88 and 1994—95 in British Columbia[J]. Age and Ageing，2000，29(3)：249—253.

⑦　Mushkin S J. Health as an Investment. Journal of Political Economy，1962(70)：129.

⑧　Becker G S. Human Capital[M]. New York：Columbia University Press（for Nat. Bur. Econ. Res.），1964.

⑨　Fuchs V R. Some economic aspects of mortality in the United States. mimeographed[M]. New York：Nat. Bur. Econ. Res.，1965.

⑩　Schultz T W. Investment in human capital[J]. American Economic Review，1961，51(1)：1—17.

多可以利用的时间,从而更多地参与生产活动,产生更大的经济效益[①]。这一理论可以更为清晰地阐述为什么较年轻死亡者的年平均医疗费用高于年纪较大的死亡者。年轻人群相对于高龄人群来说,未来期望寿命更长,因此投资于年轻人的健康,包括在终末期,所能产生的期望收益也更大。

(二)男性患者临终期费用更高

我们的研究揭示了终末期住院费用中存在的性别差异,无论是在不同年龄组还是在不同死因组中,男性费用整体高于女性,这与其他研究结果正好相反[②]。一方面由于我们没有纳入在男性中更为常见的突然死亡事件(如交通意外、工伤导致的死亡),拉高了男性群体的死亡成本。另一方面,男性(尤其是高龄男性)在临终期更倾向于在三级医疗机构住院也导致了其住院费用高于女性。这种临终前就医选择的差异有待进一步研究以揭示背后的原因。

社会观念及文化因素影响,结合健康与人力资本理论,同样可以用来解释终末期医疗费用的性别差异。在患有危急重症时,男性往往能够获得更多的医疗服务以及更高的医疗资源投入。因此,我们应当对医疗服务利用中的性别公平给予更多的关注。

(三)临终期基层就诊构成比高

事实上,与全人群相比,终末期患者更愿意选择在基层医疗机构住院,并且这种意愿随着年龄的升高而愈发强烈。然而,由于上海市基层医疗机构床位数量的限制(共 1.7 万张,占全市床位数的 14%[③]),终末期患者的医疗服务需求无法得到充分的满足。在上海,基层医疗机构的人均住院费用仅为三级医院的 30%。然而到目前为止,终末期医疗服务依旧被二三级医院所垄断。因此,加强对于基层卫生服务的资源投入、鼓励患者到基层就诊是控制医疗费用的关键环节。同时,我们应当关注基层医疗、护理以及安宁疗护服务的发展,让终末期患者能够在合适的地点获得合适的服务。

---

① Grossman M. On the concept of health capital and the demand for health[J]. Journal of Political Economy,1972,80(2):223—255.

② Blakely T,Atkinson J,Kvizhinadze G,et al. Health system costs by sex,age and proximity to death,and implications for estimation of future expenditure[J]. New Zealand Medical Journal,2014,127(1393):12—25.

③ 上海市统计局.2016 上海统计年鉴[M].北京:中国统计出版社,2016.

（四）上海市居民存在"接近死亡效应"

上海市的医疗费用存在比较明显的"接近死亡效应"。随着死亡的临近，住院服务利用以及费用均急剧上升。Felder[1]通过对 OECD 国家的研究，发现医疗费用主要被用于治疗终末期疾病，他发现，死亡前 1 个月，医疗费用急速上升，证实了距离死亡时间是影响医疗费用的一个重要因素。Seshamani 和 Gray[2]发现，由于临终前 1 年发病集中，接近死亡效应可能干扰了老龄化对医疗费用的影响。其他研究者也发现，距离死亡时间越近，产生的家庭医生费用就越高，而年龄的影响则并不显著[3]。大部分研究认为，年龄对医疗费用的影响小于距离死亡时间的影响[4][5][6]。少部分研究认为，即使控制了距离死亡时间，越来越长的期望寿命依然是医疗费用增加的一个影响因素[7]。

我们的研究发现，终末期患者临终前 1 年的住院费用中有 43%发生在死亡前 1 个月，并且该比例随着距离死亡时间的增加而降低。Lubitz[8]则发现，在 1976 年和 1988 年，临终前 1 年的医疗费用中，有 40%发生在临终前 30 天内。

从理论上来说，由于接近死亡效应与期望寿命提高的共同存在，部分年龄

---

① Felder S，Meier M，Schmitt H. Health care expenditure in the last months of life [J]. Journal of Health Economics，2000，19(5)：679—695.

② Seshamani M，Gray A. Time to death and health expenditure：An improved model for the impact of demographic change on health care costs[J]. Age and ageing. 2004，33(6)：556—561.

③ O'Neill C，Groom L，Avery A J，et al. Age and proximity to death as predictors of GP care costs：results from a study of nursing home patients[J].Health Econmics，2000，9(8)：733—738.

④ McGrail K，Green B，Barer M L，et al. Age，costs of acute and long-term care and proximity to death：Evidence for 1987—1988 and 1994—1995 in British Columbia[J]. Age and Ageing，2000(29)：249—253.

⑤ Seshamani M，Bird C E，Schuster C R. Ageing and health-care expenditure：The red herring argument revisited[J]. Health Economics，2004，13(4)：303—314.

⑥ Werblow A，Felder S，Zweifel P，et al. Population ageing and health care expenditure：A school of 'red herrings'？[J]. Health Economics，2007，16(10)：1109—1126.

⑦ Bjørner T B，Arnberg S. Terminal costs，improved life expectancy and future public health expenditure [J]. International Journal of Health Care Finance and Economics，2012，12(2)：129—143.

⑧ Lubitz J D，Rily G F. Trends in Medicare payments in the last year of life[J]. New England Journal of Medicine，1993，328(15)：1092—1097.

组的"高医疗费用"比例减少,临终费用被推迟和稀释。可以认为接近死亡效应的发现进一步厘清了老龄化造成医疗费用增长的机制,不单是由于年龄、健康状况引起,临终前医疗行为、就医模式的改变也是重要原因。

四、结语

从全人群层面来说,医疗费用随着年龄的提高而上升,但终末期住院费用却呈现出相反的规律,并且随着死亡的临近,住院费用显著增加,进一步印证了接近死亡效应的存在。但这与老龄化带来的卫生筹资压力并不矛盾,由于临终期费用的年龄别、疾病别、费用结构差异的特点,接近死亡效应与老龄化的综合作用也会呈现不同的结果。可以肯定的是,这两种效应的叠加效果给老龄化背景下的医疗费用预测带来了更大的挑战。年龄与人口总量增加(期望寿命增加)这两个因素的叠加,高医疗需求的人数总量增加,给卫生系统服务、筹资的可持续性带来考验。为了更好地保障患者需求,一方面要合理控制临终前的过度医疗费用,同时也要关注疾病负担更重的人群。

基于数据可获得性等原因,我们没有纳入在家庭及其他机构中死亡的人口,可能会导致一定的选择偏倚,高估死亡人口的医疗费用水平。

第六章

国际应对老龄化的经验

【导读】

老龄化已成为全球关注度最高的热门话题之一,也是各国不得不面对的棘手问题。多数发达国家均已进入老龄化社会,甚至部分国家即将迈入超老龄化社会,随之而来的不仅是大量老年人群的社会保障问题,同时也有相应的社会劳动力减少、社会发展进程放缓等问题。我国目前已进入老龄化社会,由于我国老年人口较多,为更好地保障这一部分人群的社会权益,让我国老年人有一个幸福安详的晚年,本章对较早进入老龄化社会的部分发达国家在应对老龄化方面开展的探索进行梳理。各个国家在不同的文化背景、卫生体制下,应对老龄化的举措有所差异,国际经验不能照搬,而且各个国家也面临自身的问题,但可借鉴其他国家的部分做法,例如,建立统一的资源调配规则,发展介护、临终服务以调整医疗服务结构,发展评估工具和系统,以需要导向提供服务等。

英国是最早进入工业化的国家,也是最早进入老龄化的国家之一。早在
20 世纪 30 年代,英国就已步入老龄化社会。到 2015 年,英国 65 岁及以上人
口占人口总数的 17.93%,85 岁及以上老人占人口总数的 2.43%。其老龄化、
高龄化程度还将进一步加深,预计到 2020 年、2030 年,65 岁及以上人口占比
将分别达到 18.86%、22.04%,85 岁及以上人口占比将分别达到 3.22%、
3.83%。老龄化伴随着人群主要疾病从急性疾病到慢性疾病、多发病、认知障
碍和长期虚弱的转变。英国在应对老年人口健康需求方面积累了丰富的经
验,而面对老龄化程度加剧的问题,英国的健康服务体系也在不断变革。

(一)英国健康服务体系概况

英国是税收型卫生服务体系的代表,国民健康服务体系(National Health
Service,NHS)自 1948 年成立以来,已发展为世界上最大的由公共资金支持的
卫生服务体系,并以其高效、公平和全面而著称。2010 年以来,英国加快了新
一轮 NHS 改革的步伐,2013 年 4 月 1 日通过了《健康和社会保健法案》,NHS
组织架构和服务提供方式也悄然变化。

1. 改革后的健康服务体系

在英国卫生部的统一管理下,改革后的 NHS 部门分为行政部门、服务购买
机构、监督规范机构和数据及证据机构、医疗服务提供机构。其中,服务购买机
构,国家层面为 NHS 委托服务委员会,是 NHS 服务委托购买的领导机构,委托
购买全国大部分初级保健和专科服务,以及地方临床委托委员会(Clinical
Commissioning Groups,CCGs)的准入。CCGs 由地方全科医生、护士及相关专业
人士组成的,负责当地医疗卫生服务规划、资源配置以及服务购买。医疗卫生服
务购买面向所有评估合格的公立、私立机构。监督规范机构对医疗卫生服务进
行质量监管、财务运行监管,反映居民的诉求;数据及证据机构中,国家卫生与临
床技术优化研究所(National Institute for Clinical Excellence,NICE)主要从循证
医学角度出发,为医务人员提供基于成本效果的临床指南和标准。医疗卫生服

务主要由地方层面提供，包括初级保健（社区医疗，Primary Care）、二级医疗（医院服务，Secondary Care）和社会照顾服务（Social Care）三个部分。国家层面购买的医疗服务，一般是地方层面提供动力不足、统筹能力不够的服务，如罕见病的治疗、军队医疗服务等，由国家统一购买，扩大风险池。具体如图 6-1 所示。

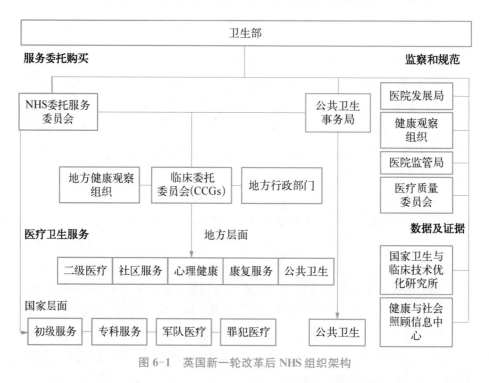

图 6-1   英国新一轮改革后 NHS 组织架构

2. 健康筹资及分配模式

2014 年，英国卫生总费用占 GDP 的 9.12%，其中 83.14% 来自广义政府卫生支出，主要是税收收入。卫生部根据卫生事项的优先顺序提出总体预算和资金总体分配，并代表 NHS 管理大型国家级项目，如研究和发展计划、IT 项目等。医疗卫生预算由财政部和议会在支出审查时审核未来预算，批准年度开支计划。2015—2016 年度总预算为 1 165 亿英镑，其中 46 亿英镑用于资产发展。1 010 亿英镑的医疗服务购买资金核拨至 NHS 委托服务委员会，其中 320 亿元由其管理、购买国家层面的医疗卫生服务；690 亿英镑分配至地方 CCGs，由地方 CCGs 组织购买地方层面的医疗卫生服务；另有 30 亿英镑用于公共卫生服务，32 亿英镑用于教育培训。英国的医疗卫生服务支付范围和定价由英格兰 NHS 委托服务委员会和医院监管局共同制定。NHS 医疗服务机构不直接获得补助，而是通过与 CCGs 签订医疗服务协议获得收入以覆盖开支。可以看出，英国并没有为老年人单独划出一部分资金；其大部分层面由地方的 CCGs 进行分配，地方层面拥有很大的灵活性，可以根据需要调整资金。

3. 健康资金支付模式及转变

改革前，NHS 对医院服务采取合同的方式打包购买一系列服务（Block Contracts），没有考虑服务质量和效率因素[①]。过去十年间，英国医疗支付方式的改革主要是为了适应老年人慢性病多发及多种疾病并发的特点，但由于没有任何一种支付方式能满足所有的政策目标，不同的服务内容仍选择了不同的支付方式。支付方式包括打包支付（按一定范围的医疗服务内容）、按人头支付（按一定人数的医疗服务）、按服务项目支付以及按绩效支付（提供指定的符合质量的医疗服务）。打包支付仍为主导的支付方式，但在急症服务系统中增加了基于产出支付方式来减少排队等待，补充了基于绩效、最佳实践支付以提高服务质量。全科医生（General Practitioner，GP）按人头签订全科服务合同（General Medical Service）。NHS 医院主要提供专科和急诊服务，大多需要与 CCGs 签订服务合同，病人一般要通过 GP 的转诊才能进入。医院服务的资金基于 CCGs 分配公式来核定，核定的基础是服务人口数量，人均权重更多地考量所在地医疗卫生服务需要，老年人口比例就是资金分配考虑的重要因素，在其他条件相同的情况下，老年人口较多的地区人均资金分配额较高。

多种支付方式并存可能给机构间协作、整合型医疗服务提供带来障碍。对于支付方式的效果评价，除了要分析支付方式对医疗行为的影响外，更重要的是关注政策目标是否实现。未来英国的支付方式改革将转向支持新的医疗护理综合模式，更好地应对老龄化健康服务需求。包括以下措施：首先，支持综合健康服务模式，如集多学科专科服务、初级保健、急症救治为一体的服务，按人头支付包括初级保健、二级医疗、社区服务、精神卫生和社会照护在内的服务；其次，支持急救网络发展，委员会基于服务能力、服务产出和服务质量对提供方进行支付，分担服务提供者的风险，确保患者在正确的环境、合适的时间接受所需服务；再次，优先支持高质量的专科、护理服务。

（二）英国健康服务模式及整合型服务探索

1. 英国老年人健康服务的一般模式

英国的健康服务体系包括初级卫生保健、医院服务、临终照护等。

---

① 　Farrar S，Sussex J，Yi D，et al. National evaluation payment by results：Report to the department of Health[R].UK：2007：6—8.

（1）初级卫生保健

GP 向每位患者提供免费初级卫生保健服务，作为"守门人"的角色，负责在病重或有特殊需要时进行住院相关服务的转诊。初级卫生保健与公共卫生服务整合后，强化了疾病预防职能。

（2）医院服务

包括急诊、专科门诊及检查、手术治疗和住院护理等[①]，提供医院服务的健康服务机构大多需要与 PCTs 签订为当地居民提供医疗服务的合同；由于英国有比较严格的"守门人"首诊制度，病人一般要通过 GP 转诊才能进入医院服务体系。

（3）临终照护

主要为临终者（Terminally Ⅲ）提供关怀照护服务。这类服务既有机构式照护，也有家庭式照护，即由专业人员为住在家里的临终老人提供家庭照护。政府提出 2015—2020 年舒缓疗护/临终关怀总体目标和六大愿景，包括尊重个体差异、确保服务公平可及、提高舒适度和幸福感、合作医疗护理、发动所有员工和全社会的力量予以帮助。要达到这些愿景，必须在多方面打好基础，包括针对个体服务的规划、教育和培训、共同设计、数据和信息、信息共享、7/24全天候可及、丧亲支持和领导力等。

此外，英国引进社会照护，由家人、朋友、邻居、社区志愿者为老年人提供居家服务，政府会对提供服务的人员提供一定的补贴；也可以由专业工作人员提供，主要通过社区服务设施，托老所、老年人公寓等资源对老人进行开放式的照顾，使其在熟悉的环境中获得养老服务。为帮助长期处于孤独与隔离状态的老人改善生活质量，英国就业养老金部于 2010 年 11 月提供 100 万资金，帮助最有可能长期处于孤独与隔离状态的老人，提升他们的生活积极性和独立性，并使其在退休后能够积极融入社会；并在 2010—2012 年与地方政府联合实施了"老年幸福"计划，主要推动地方议会通过提升社会服务水平满足老年人各方面需求，从而改善老年人生活质量。

英国的医疗卫生服务与社会服务分属卫生部和地区政府两个不同的部门管理，历史上存在服务不连贯的问题[②]。同时 NHS 服务体系又涉及全科服务、社区卫生服务、精神卫生服务、医院急诊服务等多个体系和服务机构，服

---

① 刘纯，尚尔宁，邵志高.英国医院临床药学服务模式初探[J].药学服务与研究,2015,15(5)：347—350.

② 谢春艳，金春林，王贤吉.英国整合型保健发展经验及启示[J].中国卫生资源,2015,18(1)：71—74.

务体系在多个机构之间割裂且呈碎片化,导致服务衔接困难、服务重复和资源浪费。英国探索的面向老年人的整合医疗服务大多关注健康风险等级、患者管理、准入及转出服务。"整合"包括机构、组织、系统、模式之间的协同与合作,跨越初级卫生保健、医院服务、社区照护服务的界限,推动与健康相关的各种服务的有效衔接与融合。整合型保健作为英国卫生战略规划的一部分,已成为提高国民健康和福利水平的重要基石。

2. 英国各地区整合型服务探索

(1) 英格兰南部托贝的整合医疗实践及效果

托贝(Torbay)整合医疗是英国早期整合医疗试点之一,在托贝模式中,相关部门建立一系列的联合协议、框架和策略,整合老年人服务相关的内容、经费预算,统筹预算服务于当地约 3 万居民。建立卫生和社会服务相协调的综合服务团队,共同提供保健服务;支持符合标准的病人早日从医院出院,综合服务团队帮助老年人在社区独立生活。通过整合医疗实践,医院质量、绩效和财务方面都有所改善,托贝每日平均被占用的床位数由 1998—1999 年的 750 个下降至 2009—2010 年的 502 个,65 岁及以上人口的急救床位使用率是该地区最低的。2003—2008 年,75 岁及以上人群的急救床位使用量下降 24%,85 岁及以上人群下降 32%。

(2) 伦敦卡姆登区的综合健康服务模式

伦敦卡姆登综合护理服务建立了医疗和社会照顾多学科团队,包括心理健康服务、社会服务、当地全科医生、综合初级保健团队和医院共同组成的中央枢纽多学科团队。在服务路径上,强调以需要为导向。卡姆登开发了 eFrailty index(eFI),用于分析初级保健记录数据,以便根据依赖程度、风险层级对老年人的健康状况做出正确的评价,判断医疗需要属于急症治疗还是常规护理。eFI 脆弱等级分为四级,其中,适度脆弱(eFI score 0~0.12)指没有或几乎没有长期病症的人,这个群体可独立地生活;轻度脆弱(eFI score 0.13~0.24)指可能需要在个人日常生活中(如理财、购物、交通等)得到帮助的老年人;中度脆弱(eFI score 0.25~0.36)指进行户外活动有困难或者行动不便者,需要一些帮助,如洗漱、穿衣;严重脆弱(eFI score>0.36)指经常依靠个人护理而且有一系列长期病症、多发病的人群,这类群体中有的人病情稳定,有的不稳定,并有可能在 6~12 个月内死亡。

根据服务需要,将患者诊疗路径分为几类。其一是急症治疗,首先在全科医生诊所治疗,如果病情无好转,然后以急性病住院。其二是要综合住院,则立即安排住院，完成急性治疗后转移到常规护理服务。其三是常规护理，首先评估是适用于个案管理还是日常定期护理。个案管理则首先需要评估老年人的风险现状，分诊进入适当层级的多学科团队个案管理；适合日常定期护理的老年人则进入综合护理服务，提供全科医院、社区护理、门诊、心脏健康护理、志愿部门、成人社会服务等综合定期监护服务。具体如图 6-2 所示。

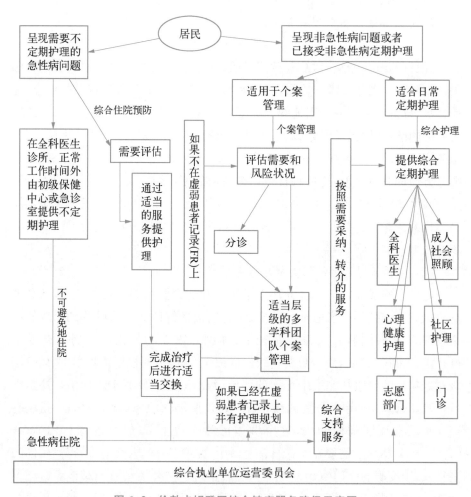

图 6-2 伦敦卡姆登区综合健康服务路径示意图

（3）伦敦西区的分级护理模式

伦敦西区为医疗与社会照顾需要制定护理规划，护理员和患者家属平等参与护理决策。根据老年人口健康状况对护理模式进行分级：65 岁以上，基本健康,为 0 级;65 岁以上,患有 1 种慢性疾病,且疾病得到良好管理,为 1 级;65 岁以上,患有 2 种或以上慢性疾病,并有心理、医疗/社会照顾需要,为 2 级;65 岁以上,患有 3 种或以上慢性疾病,并有心理、医疗/社会照顾需要,为 3 级。对不同级别人员进行差别化护理服务:0 级老年人可以在家中通过用户或者护理员自我管理,1 级老年人由医疗提供连锁协会(负有临床责任并承担实名问责的全科医生)管理,2 级老年人则在全科医生由个案管理人(负有临床责任并承担实名问责的全科医生)管理,3 级老年人则在北/南护理枢纽由护理识别服务团队提供服务。通过以上方式来为 65 岁以上老人定向增加自我护理资源、护理员参与和初级保健。护理枢纽主要由以下构成:(a) 护理之家团队:主要包括诊断、药店、社会工作者、志愿部门、职业疗法专家、心理健康、其他关联医疗服务、风险专家等各领域专家、老年病学家、理疗等;(b) 临床负责人:包括管理负责人、医疗提供连锁协会高级管理人、高级个案管理人;(c) 个案管理人:由全科医生、护理识别服务(紧急护理)、医疗提供连锁协会构成,是枢纽的拓展角色。

(4) 剑桥临终关怀服务模式

剑桥整合了初级卫生保健、二级医疗和社区卫生服务,为区域内居民提供临终关怀服务。当地各个健康服务相关机构广泛使用"临终关怀计划工具"(End of Life Care Planning Tools),帮助患者选择适宜的临终期地点。2011 年对该试点的评估显示,该地区所有登记在册的临终患者中,90% 的患者在建议的地点度过生命最后一段旅程。

(5) 伦敦西北区的全系统整合型服务模式

伦敦西北区(Northwest London)的 8 个 CCGs 地区,来自卫生、社会服务和志愿者行业的 30 多个组织机构结合在一起,开发了全系统项目(见图 6-3),此举将老年人整合医疗系统发展计划从试点阶段推进到整个系统实施阶段,核心是把全科医生作为组织和协调保健服务的核心。

(6) 牛津郡整合全系统整合模式

牛津郡位于英格兰南部,其整合医疗主要举措如下。

第一,搭建整合型的管理和治理架构。在区域范围内建立一系列的联合协议、框架和策略,整合老年人服务相关的内容、经费预算,合作范围覆盖了所有医疗卫生、养老机构服务、居家服务、辅助设备、康复服务、跌倒预防服务等。

第二,确定共同的政策目标,使不同部门和机构形成长期稳定的合作。牛津郡的政策目标包括:让更多的老年人在社区中维持安全、健康和独立自主

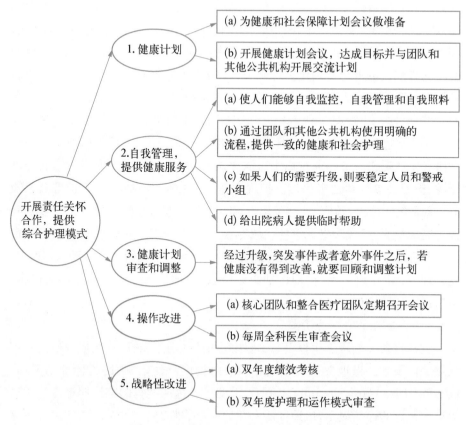

图6-3 伦敦西北区整合型服务运作模式

的生活；提高县域内服务的可及性；通过提高预防保健和早期干预措施，减少老年人急诊服务入院的数量；在急诊和住院服务中，减少因为延迟出院浪费的时间和费用。

第三，横向整合基础设施。卫生和社会服务分散于不同的设施中，为了提高老年人服务对当地居民的可及性，基础设施建设和服务设计上就考虑到卫生和社会两方面的服务，使不同的服务尽可能地共享同一地点。

第四，在评估的基础上建立医疗服务路径。利用风险分层工具（Risk Stratification Tool）识别风险人群和重点人群。重点人群由多学科服务团队再次评估，根据需要评估结果对不同人群分别建立整合型的服务路径，制定具体的诊断、服务及转诊标准；加强风险人群和重点人群的疾病预防和健康管理，避免不必要的住院。开展服务成效和人群健康结果评价，根据评价结果对服务路径不断改进。

第五，整合人力资源和工作管理。多部门合作最大的挑战之一就是如何使不同职业特征、工作特点、薪酬待遇的人员有效合作。牛津郡的主要做法是对业务进行规范化，将薪酬待遇标准化，对团队成员进行整合服务相关培训，达成团队成员之间的理解。此外，对于影响老年人的重大问题设置了重点专项，如预防跌倒专项、康复保健专项。

（三）英国健康服务体系改革的经验及启示

1. 拥有统一的组织文化和强大的系统领导力

英国是典型的高福利国家，提供从"摇篮"到"坟墓"的保障，起源于贝弗里奇社会保障计划，保障所有居民的基本生活和健康权益，注重公平和需要导向。在此文化影响下，社会各界对于保障老年人健康服务具有很强的认同度。在共同的政策目标下，民政、规划等部门和机构形成了较为紧密的合作关系，部分探索建立了相关部门联合协议、框架和策略，整合老年人服务相关的内容、经费预算，合作范围覆盖所有医疗卫生、养老机构服务、居家服务、辅助设备、康复服务、跌倒预防服务等。

卫生部系统本身具有强大的领导力。公立医疗资源占 90% 以上，由卫生行政部门统一管理。在资金管理上，NHS 临床委托委员会制定医疗资金分配的公式，并管理地方 CCGs 的准入，把控资金分配总原则，并将老年人口比例作为分配系数；约 60% 的资金由地方 CCGs 进行分配，给予地方根据实际需要进行资金分配的灵活性。管理方式和支付模式支持整合型服务。各地可因地制宜探索应对老龄化的健康服务模式，支付方式改革将转向支持新的医疗护理综合模式及多系统协作服务。

2. 基于需要，以 GP 为纽带开展整合型健康服务

英国整合型医疗服务主要围绕服务利用者的需要提供协同性服务，整合预防服务和治疗服务，树立"以患者为根本，以健康为中心"的服务理念，强化社区对老年居民疾病的早期预警及有效防控。英国各个地区在不同层面进行了整合型健康服务试点，在宏观层面建立政府部门间的协作机制，统筹预算分配；在微观层面从医疗、护理、临终关怀等不同角度探索整合的模式。得益于英国强大的初级保健服务力量、高质量的全科医生队伍，全科医生在整合医疗体系中发挥了核心的作用，不仅负责初级保健、疾病管理，更是患者分诊、不同机构间协作的纽带。整合型的健康服务以初级卫生保健和公共卫生服务为主导，与慢性病为主的疾病谱的特点相适应，实现了一级预防、二级预防，降低了

疾病治疗的负担。在服务提供过程中，推行多学科综合治疗（Multi-Disciplinary Team，MDT）模式，根据老年人个体制定有针对性的、个性化的服务包，由固定的多学科服务团队负责提供服务并进行健康管理，满足老年人身体相对虚弱、共患疾病比例高的医疗需要特点，并从社会学角度从精神、心理上给予支持。

上海市建立了包括村卫生室、乡镇卫生院、社区卫生服务机构的基本医疗卫生服务网络，但无论是资源配置还是诊疗模式，仍以急性期疾病治疗为主，服务体系中的预防功能、老年人慢性病的管理还比较薄弱，需进一步加强基层的资源整合能级、人员培养，规范医疗服务、建立"以人为中心"的生物—心理—社会医学模式。考虑到老年人共患疾病比例高、多器官症状并发的特点，为了保证疾病得到安全有效的治疗，多个医疗卫生机构、卫生技术人员间应该高度合作，而且使用的技术、药品应适宜、协同。医院需进一步发展 MDT 服务，由多学科专家共同为老年疾病会诊，为老年患者就诊提供综合的诊疗服务。

3. 以数据、分析工具为支持的决策体系

实时、准确地应对老年人健康服务需要是实现分类管理、整合服务的基础。英国注重健康、医疗数据整合和知识管理平台的搭建，充分发挥高校、研究机构、企业的力量，建立数据驱动的健康需要评估。在高校（如帝国理工学院数据科学研究所）和健康维护组织开展大数据挖掘，支撑健康服务发展。各地对健康信息进行采集、标化，并将这些信息充分应用于管理。如伦敦中区西北区信托医院（CNWL）通过对健康服务机构的数据采集，构建生产系统、临床系统和管理系统的数据集成平台。首先，整合数据可实现对各医疗团队和医疗机构质量及绩效的定期监测。其次，大数据是准确评估老年人的健康服务需要的前提。英国已经开发了多种风险预测工具，并在NHS组织中得到广泛应用。如卡姆登地区的 eFrailty Index（eFI）、伦敦西北区的护理评估体系、剑桥的临终关怀计划工具、牛津郡的风险分层工具。最后，根据需要提供服务的体系有效支持了健康服务资源在不同老年群体中的合理分配，促进了卫生体系总体绩效的提高。

近年来，上海市医疗卫生机构的信息化水平逐步提高，下一步重点是将这些"信息孤岛"联结起来，利用平台数据开展决策分析，实现对高风险群体的有效管理，加强医疗质量监管，使资源得到更合理配置。

二、日本应对老龄化的经验及对中国的启示[①]

(一)日本老龄化的趋势及变化

根据联合国对老龄化社会的定义,凡 65 岁及以上老年人口占总人口比例达到 7%以上或 60 岁及以上老年人口在总人口中比重超过 10%时,该区域即属于老龄化国家或地区。日本自 1970 年进入老龄化社会以来,以极快的增速在 24 年后(即 1994 年)达到了 14%的 65 岁及以上老年人口比例,而同样的老龄化进程,美国用了 72 年,英国用了 46 年。截至 2015 年,日本的 65 岁及以上老年人口比例为 26.7%,位居世界第一,成为全世界老龄化程度最高的国家。日本厚生劳动省在 2016 年白皮书中对日本的未来人口发展趋势进行预测,预计到 2060 年,日本 65 岁及以上老年人口数为 3 464 万人,老年人口比例将达到 39.9%,平均每2.5人中有 1 人为老年人。而相对的劳动人口与青少年人口自 1990 年开始便一直保持下降趋势,并将在 2060 年分别降至 50.9%和9.1%(见图 6-4)。

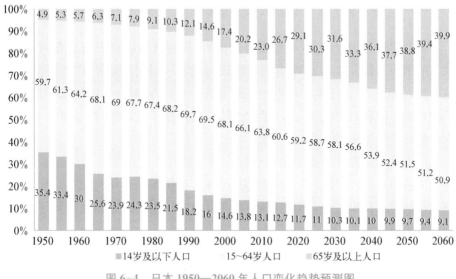

图 6-4　日本 1950—2060 年人口变化趋势预测图

① 本节所有内容均来源于日本厚生劳动省官方网站(http://www.mhlw.go.jp/)。

　　因此,随着日本社会老龄化进程的不断推进,年轻人对老年人的抚养比也在不断下降。2015 年,1 位 65 岁及以上老年人口由 2.1 位劳动人口进行支撑,这一数值将于 2050 年下降到 1.2,并长期保持在这一较低水平(见图 6-5)。

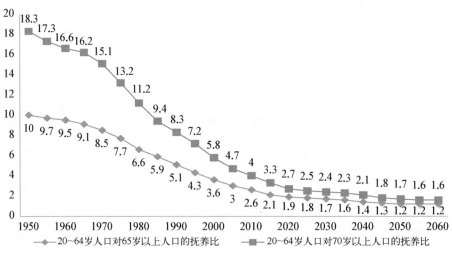

图 6-5　日本 1950—2060 年老年人口抚养比变化趋势预测图

(二)日本老年人医疗及介护保障体系

　　第二次世界大战后,日本社会百废待兴,政府鼓励国民积极生育,日本二战后的第一次婴儿生育高峰也相应出现,并被日本国民统称为"团块世代"。这一代人作为 20 世纪推动日本经济腾飞的主要动力,被日本国民视作日本经济的脊梁。随着时光流逝,团块世代也陆续退休并步入老年时代,对日本老年人口的社会保障提出了挑战。

　　日本社会保障体系主要由社会保险体系和社会救助体系共同组成,社会保险体系包括医疗保险、年金保险、失业保险、工伤保险和介护保险,社会救助体系包括生活保护和社会福利,其中社会福利进一步细分为儿童福利、残障福利和老年福利。

　　日本的社会保险为强制保险,由各级政府机关或社会团体作为保险人,以保险费作为经费,对被保险人提供保险服务(见表 6-1)。其中,进入职场工作的人员相较其他日本国民享受相对较高的保障水平,且从被保险人范围可以看出,日本社会保险中以家庭为单位的色彩较为浓重,体现了更高的社会共济能力。

表 6-1　日本社会保险制度概况

保险类型	种　类	类　别	保险人	被保险人	保险给付	给付形式
年金保险	地区保险	国民年金	国家	20～60 岁国民	退休	金钱给付
	职场保险	厚生年金	国家	职场工薪人员、公务员等	由于残疾而无法工作者；配偶死亡	
医疗保险	职场保险	健康保险（组合）	健康保险协会	工作时间超过 30 周的工薪人员；由工薪人员所抚养的人员	由于工作以外的原因而生病、受伤	以医疗服务给付为主,金钱给付为辅
		共济组合保险	共济组合			
	地区保险	国民健康保险	市町村政府	自营人员；未参与工作者		
		后期高龄老年人医疗保险	后期高龄老年人医疗地域联合	75 岁及以上国民		
工伤保险	职场保险		国家	所有劳动人员	由于工作原因而生病、受伤	以医疗服务和金钱给付为主,福利服务给付为辅
失业保险			国家	工作时间超过 20 周的所有劳动者	想工作但实际没有在工作的失业	金钱给付
介护保险	地区保险		市町村政府	在各市町村拥有住所的 40 岁以上人员	被认定为要支援、要介护状态	福利服务给付为主,医疗服务给付为辅

1. 医疗保障制度

（1）全民医疗保障制度

日本在建立医疗保险时即体现了强烈的人人享有医疗卫生服务并共担社会风险的中心思想。日本医疗保险通过立法,确认了每一位公民的参保义务,医疗保险基金来源于保险费，除却被保险人需缴纳保险费外，其供职的机构也需一同负担，此外对于收入较低的人员，根据其收入水平，可进行保险费用的减免，并由国家财政或地方公共团体对减免部分进行支付。该保险制度以较低的保险费用水平建立了全社会共同承担风险的基金，并充分体现了日本社会崇尚的自立、自助的生活方式。

日本的医疗保险主要可分为四种模式：一是由企业上班族为主要构成的健康保险，根据企业规模可分为由大企业上班族构成的健康保险组合（截至2016年的被保险人约为2 870万人，下同）以及由中小企业上班族构成的由全国健康保险协会提供的协会健保（被保险人约为3 550万人）；二是由公务员参加的共济组合，被保险人约为870万人；三是由其他各类人群加入的国民健康保险（包括个体户、临时工、依靠年金生活的人等），由各地的市町村政府进行运营，保险额会根据地区、年收入等因素进行调整和浮动，该类型被保险人约为3 600万人；四是后期高龄老年人医保制度，共计有参保人约1 660万人。

（2）后期高龄老年人医疗保险制度

日本在2008年4月建立了针对75岁及以上高龄老年人和65～74岁残疾老年人的后期高龄老年人医保制度，当日本老年人年满75周岁或年满65～74周岁但被认定为残疾（以下统称为后期高龄老年人），则由原来所参加的医疗保险统一转移至该保险进行保障。这一面向后期高龄老年人的医疗保险制度，旨在应对老龄化社会对传统医疗保险（主要指国民健康保险）所带来的挑战，降低老年人的医疗保险支付水平，提高社会对后期高龄老年人的关注和共济水平，以确保后期高龄老年人对医疗卫生服务的公平可及性。该保险制度由日本47个地区联合团体作为主要的运营主体，根据被保险人的收入水平，由市町村政府征收保险费，由于后期高龄老年人的收入来源大部分为养老金，因此大部分人的保险费征收方式为直接从养老金中进行扣除。为了进一步减轻地区联合团体运营后期高龄老年人医保制度的财务风险，国家及都道府县政府也对该保险制度给予了一定的保障并建立了风险分担机制。

截至2016年，后期高龄老年人保险基金为15兆日元，全部保险费用的50%为公费负担，40%为其他医疗保险对该保险制度的风险共济，剩余的10%为后期高龄老年人支付的保险费用。另根据最新的后期高龄老年人医保制度全国统计显示，2015年该保险参保人共发生医疗费用15.1兆日元，相比2014年增长了4.4%。由于日本设置了自负费用封顶线制度，实际操作中给付率高于制度所设定的报销比例。2015年通过保险基金给付医疗费用14.0兆日元，给付率达到 92.2%。即使是按照法律规定应自负 30% 的被保险人（仍从事社会生产或拥有养老金以外的生活来源），其给付率亦达到了 81.3%。从人均医疗费来看，2015 年，后期高龄老年人医保制度的参保人年人均医疗费用为 94.9 万日元，与 2014 年相比增长了 1.8%。

后期高龄老年人医保制度依据的《高龄老年人医疗确保法》不仅仅是将后期高龄老年人从整个医保体系中剥离，形成了独立的运转体系，还对 65～74 岁老年人的医保筹资比例进行了调整；即在政府层面，不同类型的基金统筹使用，职场保险、国民健康保险基金按一定比例对 65～74 岁参保人员的费用进行支付，平衡了不同类别保险基金的实际支出。具体来说，由于日本职场的退休年龄一般为 65 周岁，因此该年龄段的老年人多属于国民健康保险的保障范围。为了减轻国民健康保险的运营压力，在建立后期高龄老年人医保制度的同时，将国民健康保险对该年龄段老年人医疗费用的支付比例由原来的 80% 降低到 35%，而将健保组合、共济组合和协会健保的支付比例由原来的 20% 提高到了 65%。

值得一提的是，由于日本存在被雇佣者所抚养的家属属于被雇佣者所在保险的保障范畴的现象，而年长的父母亦属于这一范畴，因此后期高龄老年人医保制度的推出导致部分原先属于被抚养者而免费享受医疗保障的老年人必须缴纳额外的保险费用，引起了部分国民的不满。

（3）筹资

① **保险费**。日本的医疗保险费征收方式，根据保险制度的保障对象不同，可主要分为两类，即雇佣者保险（包括健康保险组合、协会健保和共济组合）和国民健康保险。雇佣者保险的保险费是按照该雇佣者每月工资的一定比例进行计算，业主和被雇佣者各付一半。因为按照工资比例计算保险费，因此对工资的计算有根据社会总体经济水平所划定的上下限值。除工资之外，被雇佣者每年发放的奖金也需要按照同样比例缴纳保险费，同样定有上限值。值得一提的是，被雇佣者如果是医疗保险参保人，则由其所抚养的家属都可以作为被抚养者的身份受保，且由于被雇佣者保险费仅按照该雇佣者收入的一定比例进行计算，与被抚养者人数无关，因此，对于保险者来说，这些被抚养者是否依据法律具有享受医疗保险的资格，需要经过相关部门的严格审查。对国民健康保险来说，该保险费是根据全家人的总收入比例，再加上全家人数的每个人的基本定额进行计算。同时，政府规定每个家庭一年所缴纳的保险费额具有上限，无论家庭收入和人数多少均不能超过该上限。

② **基金状况**。各类保险制度的基金状态根据参保人员和保费的缴纳水平而具有差异。例如健康保险组合的参保人主要为大企业的上班族，与其他保险相比，具有参保人员年龄结构低、人均医疗费用低、平均收入较高等特点，因此该保险的基金总体较为稳定；国民健康保险的参保人主要为个体户、临时工、依靠年金收入生活且未满 75 岁的退休人员等，与其他保险相比，具有参保人员年龄结构较高、人均医疗费用较高、平均收入较低等特点，因此该保险的基金总体处于较不稳定的状态，特别是近年来有较多人员由于退休等原因由其他保险类型转为国民健康保险，因此基金总体情况较为严峻。日本为了调整这类由于参保人员不同而造成的保险基金不稳定的情况，针对 65～74 岁的老年人制定了前期老年人财政调整制度，且特别对相对其他保险类型更为脆弱的国民健康保险实行了低收入者强化对策，基于低收入者实际数量进行了财政转移支付。此外，由于后期高龄老年人医保制度建设而导致国民的不满，政府开始计划对该制度的废除工作，将其与国民健康保险合并，回到最初的医疗保险体系，并进一步强化国民健康保险的基金稳定程度，对《国民健康保险法》进行修正，明确了自 2018 年起，国民健康保险的责任运营主体将由市町村政府改变为都道府县政府，而市町村政府继续执行包括资格管理、保险费征收等具体事务，以此确保国民健康保险基金的财务平衡。

（4）医疗费用

① **诊疗报酬**。对日本医疗保险的参保人来说，仅需在医疗机构就诊时出示保险证，就可以享受医疗保险，且在结账时按照比例支付医疗费用的自负部分即可，余下的医疗费用由医疗机构直接与保险机构进行交涉。医疗机构根据对每一位患者进行的医疗服务获得诊疗报酬，由医疗机构每月将上一月开展的医疗服务形成具有诊疗明细的申请单提交至由保险机构成立的地区审查支付机构（国民健康保险为国民健康保险团体联合会，其他保险类型为社会保险医疗费支付基金），由该机构的诊疗报酬审查委员会经过审查后对余下的诊疗报酬进行支付。若在审查过程中发现不当的医疗服务申请，则诊疗报酬将被拒绝支付。若多次发现，则该医生或医疗机构将被处分。一旦被拒绝支付，则该申请将被视为无效申请，则此前向患者收取的诊疗费用也将成为不正当收益，应向该患者退款，并详细列出退款明细。此外，日本法律规定，各服务项目的诊疗报酬应每两年进行一次调整，以符合日本社会经济的发展。同时，通过调整诊疗报酬标准，有导向性地提高适宜技术的报酬水平，降低不适宜技术的报酬标准，以此规范诊疗行为。

② **患者负担。** 在日本,无论患者参加何种医疗保险,其自负比例仅与年龄及年收入水平相关。一般情况下,日本医疗保险的患者负担比例为全部医疗费用的 30%,学龄前儿童为 20%,70 岁及以上但未到 75 岁的老年人根据其年收入分为 20% 或 30%,而 75 岁及以上老年人则根据其所得收入可分为10% 或 30%(主要取决于该老年人是否尚在工作)。为了避免患者在整个医疗过程中负担过重,日本设有专门的高额疗养费制度,即当患者的月自负医疗费用(不包含住院餐费等)超过一定限额时,超过的部分将由保险进行支付,该支付上限根据年龄进行区别。此外,当医疗费用和介护费用的自负部分合计超过一定限额时,也设有相类似的高额医疗、高额介护合计疗养费制度。

③ **变化趋势。** 日本政府承担的医疗费用支出近年来呈现上升趋势,2014年达到了 40.8 兆日元,而后期高龄老年人医疗费用占政府医疗费用总支出的比例虽然在 2003 年时由于政府政策调整,将后期高龄老年人的年龄由 70 岁调整到了 75 岁而产生了些微的下降,但近年来仍保持了逐渐上升的趋势(见图 6-6)。

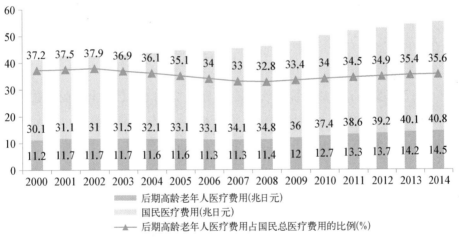

图 6-6　2002—2014 年日本后期高龄老年人政府医疗费用支出情况

(5)服务提供

日本医疗服务提供体系以公私并存为主,且私立医疗机构在日本医疗服务系统中居主体地位。在患者就医方面没有强制性基层首诊制度,患者可根据个人意愿自由就诊。

① **医疗机构。** 截至 2015 年,日本共有 178 212 家医疗机构,其中医院

8 480家,一般诊所 100 995 家,牙科诊所 68 737 家。根据产权进行分类,私立医疗机构 172 253 家,占全部医疗机构的 96.66%,其中医院 6 924家,一般诊所 96 871 家,牙科诊所 68 458 家。在日本,拥有 20 张及以上床位的医疗机构被定义为医院,20 张以下或没有床位的医疗机构为一般诊所,因此,诊所被进一步细分为有床诊所(7 961 家)和无床诊所(93 034 家)。根据 2014 年《医疗法》中修订的内容,对有床诊所的职责进行了明确的规定,主要承担着出院病人到正常生活间无缝连接的作用(包括康复期必要的医疗服务提供、居家医疗服务提供等)、急性疾病的必要医疗服务提供以及地区医疗服务体系的支援等。历年统计数据显示,与 1996 年相比,2014 年日本的无床诊所增加了 1.4 倍,有床诊所则减少了 60%。

② **病床数**。统计数据显示,日本 2015 年共拥有床位数 1 673 669 张,其中医院床位数为 1 565 968 张,一般诊所为 107 626 张,牙科诊所为 75 张。从产权归属来看,医院的所有床位中,私立医疗机构床位占比达到 71.21%(1 115 144 张);一般诊所的私立医疗机构床位占比则达到了 95.51%(102 792 张)。截至 2014 年,日本的每万人口病床数地区差异较大。最高为高知县,每万人口拥有 248.2 张床位;最低为神奈川县,每万人口拥有 81.5 张床位。此外,日本的平均住院日与每万人口病床数呈现了基本一致的状态,平均住院日最长为高知县的 48.8 天,最短为神奈川县的 23.0 天。

③ **医师数**。日本相关统计数据显示,截至 2014 年,日本全国医师数量为 31.1 万人,除去死亡等原因保持在每年 4 000 人左右的增长幅度。相较 1984 年,其每万人口医师数由 15.1 人上升到了 24.5 人,增长了 1.3 倍(见图 6-7)。

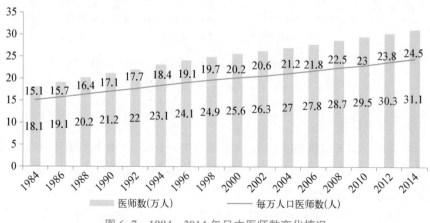

图 6-7　1984—2014 年日本医师数变化情况

2. 介护保险制度

在日本介护保险体系建立前,针对老年人的社会保障制度主要有依据《老人福祉法》建立的老年人福利制度和依据《老人保健法》建立的老年人医疗制度。然而,由于制度本身协同能力有待进一步提高,此外,随着日本高龄老年人数量的不断增加,老年人对于医疗服务和介护服务的需求日益上涨,对于老年人福利制度来说,存在制度已不能完全保障老年人的全部需求,同时社会力量也难以参与到福利服务的体系中等问题。而对于老年人医疗制度来说,也存在介护设施不完备,由于对介护服务的需求导致的社会性入院增加,医疗保险负担较大,以及人均居室面积狭小,入住服务利用者缺乏隐私,疗养环境有待进一步改善等问题。因此,日本政府决定引入社会保险制度,导入以服务利用者为中心的新型服务形式,同时将介护的部分从医疗保险制度中剥离以逐渐消减社会性入院情况,并在制度建设之初就以社会办机构作为服务最主要的提供方。

(1) 筹资

介护保险由日本1都1道2府43县政府下辖的市町村及特别区政府作为保险人,对辖区内拥有居所的住民(包括外国人)进行保险,被保险人按照年龄可分为65岁及以上老年人口的1号被保险人和40岁及以上未满65岁的2号被保险人。无论是否申请介护服务,被保险人自40岁开始按照收入比例(包括养老年金收入)终生向市町村政府缴纳介护保险金。

在介护保险费缴纳方面,1号被保险人与2号被保险人缴纳标准不同。1号被保险人的缴费金额取决于个人年收入及居住地区制定的"基准额"。日本全国以地区为单位以介护保险财政规划期为周期对基准额进行计算,根据本地区的老年人口数推算出此后3年本地区介护服务的需求量,从而推导出介护保险的估算支付额及平均每人应支付的费用,因此基准额可看作是一种"预算额"。因为1号被保险人以退休老年人为主,因此大部分人的保险费从他们的养老金中按每两月进行扣除。若1号被保险人为低保待遇人员或没有养老年金等情况,可通过缴费单、银行转账等方式每月进行缴纳。2号被保险人的缴纳标准则是根据本人的收入和参加的医疗保险种类(职场保险或国民健康保险),分别按照全国统一的医疗保险费率和介护保险费率进行计算,并从每月收入中进行扣除。若2号被保险人由于失业、提前退休等情况而属于国民健康保险保障范围时,则当地政府会根据本人的收入状况及相关保险的保险费率计算本人的缴纳额度,并通知其前往银行等进行缴纳。

（2）费用

当被保险人产生介护费用时,除却被保险人自负的10%（收入达到一定水平以上的被保险人为20%,该支付判断标准随国家经济水平进行动态调整,目前标准为本人总收入达到160万日元以上,同一家庭的1号被保险人"年金收入＋其他收入总额"单身者达到280万日元或2人以上家庭达到346万日元以上)外,另90%由介护保险基金承担,具体费用支付比例主要由两部分组成,分别为国民缴纳的保险费和政府税收各占一半。其中税收的部分由国家政府、都道府县政府、市町村政府按比例承担,当支付服务为居家养老服务时,比例分别为25%、12.5%、12.5%,当支付服务为机构养老服务时,比例分别为20%、17.5%、12.5%,保险费的部分则为1号被保险人所交的保险费约占22%,2号被保险人所交的保险费约占28%。2016年,1号被保险人的保险费支付额度总计2.1兆日元,2号被保险人的保险费支付额度总计2.8兆日元,而全部的介护保险费用支付额度为9.6兆日元。虽然2016年度的介护保险费用尚未正式统计公布,但根据历年变化情况来看,仍保持上升趋势（见图6-8）。

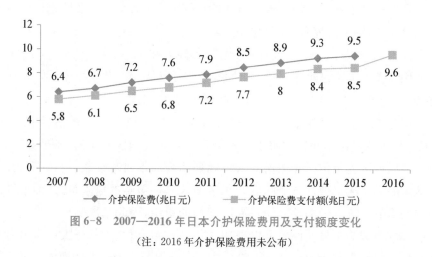

图6-8   2007—2016年日本介护保险费用及支付额度变化

（注：2016年介护保险费用未公布）

（3）服务提供

在日本,若介护保险被保险人需申请介护服务,则需要接受介护认定调查员进行的上门调查和评估。介护等级的评估主要由各市町村具体负责,都道府县主要给予财政及事务方面的支持。介护等级评估的具体程序如下。

① 被保险人向市町村政府提出要介护申请。

② 市町村派出经过培训并符合资质的评估员对申请人就74个项目进行

1次访问调查,评估采用上门评估的形式,评估的内容包括身体机能、精神及行动障碍、认知机能以及医疗处置等。评估工具为由厚生劳动省制定的、全国统一的要介护认定调查表,包括概况调查、基本调查项目和特别调查项目三个方面。评估员对调查结果进行确认后上传电脑,由已开发完成的计算程序对结果进行直接计算并得到一次判定结果。

③ 市町村委托主治医生职称以上的医生对被申请人进行健康审查,由主治医生提出健康状况意见书。

④ 市町村介护认定审查委员会根据上述调查结果和健康状况意见书进行二次认定,委员会由保健医疗福祉专家 5 人左右组成,判定内容主要是申请者的身体及情感方面的障碍程度和认知程度,并结合前项调查结果和主治医生意见书综合分析,认定最终的介护等级以及实际操作过程中是否需要花费额外的介护时间(见表 6-2),认定结果大体分为三类:一是重新调查;二是对一次判定的认定结果进行调整并同时提交调整依据;三是维持一次判定结果。申请人对认定调查结果有异议的,还可以向都道府县的介护保险审查会提出申诉。

表 6-2 日本介护服务等级、限定标准及服务内容基本要求

介护类型	等级	支付限额标准	服务基本要求
要支援 (介护预防服务)	1	52 300 日元	根据服务标准向服务利用者提供符合其个人实际需求和情况的介护预防服务,其中上门护理根据等级定额为每周提供 1~2 次,疗养管理指导每月 2 次
	2	109 500 日元	
要介护 (介护服务)	1	174 500 日元	根据服务标准向服务利用者提供符合其个人实际需求和情况的上门或机构介护服务,其中介理老人福利设施为要介护 3~5 级的老年人才可入住的设施
	2	205 000 日元	
	3	281 500 日元	
	4	322 000 日元	
	5	376 900 日元	

⑤ 由介护支援专门员上门与申请人及其家属共同商讨制定介护服务计划。

⑥ 与服务提供专业人员商讨介护服务计划,修改并开始提供介护服务。

日本介护服务的内容主要分为居家养老服务和机构养老服务。居家养老服务包括上门介护服务、生活支援服务、日托服务及养老机构的短期寄宿服务等;机构养老服务包括特别养护老人之家、老人保健设施和医院疗养病床等。

截至 2015 年，日本全国提供居家养老服务的机构数为 173 751 家；提供介护预防服务的机构数为 133 781 家；提供地区紧密型服务的机构数为 46 597 家（见表 6-3）。

表 6-3　2015 年日本居家及地区养老服务机构数　（单位：家）

机　构　类　别	机构数
居家服务机构	173 751
介护预防服务机构	133 781
地区紧密型服务机构	46 597
地区紧密型介护老人福利设施	1 901
地区紧密型服务机构	23 651
地区紧密型介护预防服务机构	21 045

在机构养老方面，截至 2015 年，日本各类型养老机构数为 16 163 家，共有从业人员 561 202 人，机构服务利用率平均在 90% 以上，入住老年人平均介护度在 3 级及以上，均符合日本介护保险法对机构养老老年人的介护度要求。其中介护疗养型医疗机构服务对象虽为要介护 1～5 级的老年人，但其平均介护度达到 4.38，均为高度要介护的老年人，可能是因为法律规定其服务内容为"基于治疗管理，向已接收治疗但需要进行长期疗养者提供看护、护理、康复等服务"，具有医疗护理和生活照料的双重属性。而由介护支援专门员制定的介护服务计划，使老年人在专业人员的协调下获得最符合其需求的介护服务，不仅使老年人仍能保持自身独立自主的生活能力，同时也提高了社会整体介护资源的利用效率（见表 6-4）。

表 6-4　2015 年日本养老服务机构及服务提供情况

机　构　类　别	机构数	从业人数	核定服务提供数	机构利用率	平均介护度
介护老人福利机构	7 551	313 363	518 273	97.4%	3.87
介护老人保健机构	7 189	201 948	368 201	89.2%	3.26
介护疗养型医疗机构	1 423	45 891	62 835	91.1%	4.38

（三）日本未来改革趋势

日本政府为了应对即将到来的超高龄社会，提出要根据地方实际情况，提高医疗和介护保险服务的效率,同时对低收入者等弱势人群进行倾斜,进一步体现了社会保障体系的社会共济作用。在服务方式上,应建立以社区为单位的综合性介护(预防)服务体系,全面推进居家养老事业,最终实现能够让所有人都充满活力且安心生活的社会。

1. 鼓励有能力的老年人继续工作

伴随着日本老龄化程度的不断提高,未来的劳动人口势必逐渐减少。2012 年,日本政府通过修订《老年人雇佣安定法》明确规定日本企业在无特殊情况下应雇佣职员一直到其 65 岁为止,同时对于有能力且有工作意愿的老年人可延长其工作时间。为了持续推进该项工作,日本政府拟在《老年人雇佣安定法》的基础上,针对 65 岁后被雇佣老年人的情况对《雇用保险法》进行修订,包括对每周工作时间、健康管理制度的导入等。而对积极开展老年人雇佣工作的企业,政府也在商讨对其进行政策方面支持的可能性。

2. 推进疾病预防和介护预防工作

为了减少要介护老年人的增加,日本社会一方面积极宣传教育日本国民保持健康生活习惯,维护自身健康,其中就包括加强国民慢性病(预防)管理;尽可能延长健康寿命;积极参与到各类社会活动中,维持正常的社会交往;对生活环境进行必要的整理;确保每日营养的摄入以及运动、休养、睡眠、口腔等生活习惯的维持和改善等。另一方面,政府以社区为单位组织社区志愿者组织等团体活动,鼓励老年人积极参与,同时增强生活中的康复性活动,完善社会保障体系对老年人的倾斜和支持,推进介护预防工作的开展以及介护服务的经营管理。

3. 推进以社区为单位的综合性服务体系

日本政府于 2013 年开始着手在全国推进社区综合性服务体系的建设工作。该体系主要是对目前日本社会医疗、介护、介护预防、住房和生活支援 5 个方面的整合,旨在建立一个更加适合老年人居家养老的社区环境和支撑体系。就医疗和介护方面来说,一是加强医疗和介护服务体系间的协同合作,主要包括确保居家养老的家庭病床服务,在社区介护的服务过程中确保医疗护理方面的需求能够被切实满足,尽可能在每个社区建立一支能够提供上门服务的医护专业团队;二是推进针对认知症患者方面的政策实施,主要包括创建适应于认知症患者的介护服务模式,在社区服务项目中加强针对认知症患者的服务内容,对社区居民加强认知症方面的健康教育,不仅让他们能够正确认识认知症,并且培养社区居民的使命感和责任感,鼓励社区居民肩负起社区内认知症患者的"监护"职责，以保证认知症患者的权益。

（四）对我国老年人社会保障体系的启示

日本作为老龄化程度位于世界前列的国家之一，在应对老龄化方面具有丰富的实践经验和教训，并一直被相关领域的专家学者所关注。本章节通过对日本老年人医疗和介护保障体系的梳理，对其发展实践进行总结。

1. 建立权责对等的老年保障体系以应对老龄化社会

日本通过建立后期高龄老年人医疗保险制度和介护保险制度，重点关注老年人群。首先，将介护服务和医疗卫生服务各自独立，明确分工，加强协同，在保证患者能够在医疗和介护间无缝衔接的同时，降低了单纯介护服务对医疗卫生服务资源的挤占。其次，提高保险基金的稳定性和持续性，加强了社会共济水平，介护保险的参保对象为 40 岁以上日本住民，强调了权利和义务之间的关系，避免将社会保障的全部压力过于集中在劳动人口，这也符合日本高龄少子化的社会现实。

2. 注重疾病和介护预防以延长老年人的健康寿命

在介护保险制度实施之初，由于老年人口和要介护老年人的急速增加以及介护服务理念的不明确，带来了介护保险支出超过预期，造成了介护保险制度严重的收支不平衡，甚至可能威胁到介护保险制度的存亡。为此，日本政府对介护保险制度实施全面改革。一是推进介护预防事业，减少或延缓要介护老年人的增长。二是严格控制介护服务的使用。由于老年人的衰老不可逆转，而日本老龄化程度只会不断加深，因此只有尽可能推迟老年人进入要介护状态的时间，才能在满足实际需求的同时控制需求快速增长，从而减少介护保险费用的支出。介护预防与疾病预防的理念相似，均是为防止后期产生大量成本支出而进行的早期干预。预防的理念不仅延长了老年人的健康寿命和自理时间，同时也提高了社会资源的配置效率。

3. 根据需求提供服务以维持老年人的自理能力

在日本介护保险制度建立之初的服务理念是尽可能地满足要介护老年人的所有需求，然而事实证明，这一理念与介护保险制度建立的目标之间存在误差。已有大量研究证明，给予老年人过度的介护服务不仅浪费了社会介护资源，还在很大程度上降低了老年人独立生活的能力，最终影响老年人的身心健康。经过系列改革后，日本在提供介护服务前需经过专业调查员的评估，如同医生给患者进行诊断一般，在经过计算机软件和专业人员对介护度进行两次判定后,还会有专业人员上门为老年人量身制定符合其需求的介护服务计划。整个过程都体现了《介护保险法》第4条"在要介护状态下进行的康复以及其他的医疗服务及福利服务均是为了增进其自身拥有的能力而提供的"的规定。也就是说,无论老年人处于什么状态,对其开展介护服务的最终目标都是为了能使该名老年人最终即使不再使用这些服务也能独立生活(虽然大部分老年人由于衰老或其他原因终身都需要依靠介护服务)。因此服务不在于多,而在于在不损害老年人自立能力的前提下是否为其当下切实需要。

4. 加强人才队伍培养以满足社会增长的服务需求

无论是医疗服务还是介护服务,均离不开由专业人员提供的服务。目前我国医养结合体系正在逐步完善,这不仅需要各部门间、各机构间加强协同合作,还需要服务团队或一线服务人员对其他学科的服务内容具有一定的了解和学习。因此,建立对医疗、介护方面服务人员的专业技能培训、继续教育机制非常重要。此外,日本对于不同服务方向和内容的专业人员均有其专业资质考试和证书,包括介护支援专门员、看护师、介护师、康复师、言语听觉师等,这不仅能够规范整个服务队伍,提高服务质量,同时也可通过国家政策的重视提高这些专业人员的社会地位,使他们有更好的职业发展规划。

三、荷兰健康体系应对老龄化的经验及对上海的启示

根据2015年"欧洲健康消费者指数(Euro Health Consumer Index,EHCI)"评选结果,荷兰医疗体系被评为欧盟年度最佳医疗体系;同时,荷兰也是2005年以来,唯一一个在欧盟医疗体系排名中始终位居前三位的国家①②。荷兰的医疗保险模式在全球范围内可谓独树一帜,其医改模式可概括为政府调控下的市场主导型,其独创的"管理型市场竞争"模式是在2006年改革后形成的,这一创新性的改革使得保险公司、医疗保健提供者和被保险人三者能够相互制约与平衡,最终使整个医疗保健市场达到自由选择、有序竞争的状态③。

---

① 戴廉.2008欧洲医疗体系,谁最令消费者满意?[J].中国医院院长,2009,Z1:35—36.

② Health Consumer Powerhouse. Euro health consumer index 2015 report[DB/CD].(2016-01-26).

③ 吴君槐.荷兰医保独树一帜[J].中国卫生,2015(4):110—111.

（一）荷兰人口老龄化情况

荷兰地处西欧，与德国、比利时接壤。其国土面积为 41 543 平方公里，拥有 1 704 万人口（2017 年）[①]。其国内生产总值（GDP）位于世界前 20 位，出口量为世界前十位[②]。荷兰的老龄化过程可以大致分为四个阶段。第一个阶段是 1900—1950 年，本阶段是荷兰人口老龄化的起步阶段。1900 年，荷兰 65 岁以上老年人口占总人口的 6.0%，1950 年上升为 7.7%，标志着荷兰人口进入老龄化阶段。第二个阶段是 1951—1990 年，荷兰进入人口老龄化快速发展阶段。本阶段，其 65 岁以上人口占总人口的比重几乎以每十年增加 1 个百分点的速度稳步上升。到 1990 年，上升到 12.8%。第三个阶段是 1991—2040 年，该阶段，荷兰人口老龄化程度急剧上升，预计在 2030—2040 年达到峰值。第四个阶段则是 2041—2060 年，将是其人口老龄化的高峰平台阶段[③]。

（二）荷兰健康保健体系

荷兰健康保健体系主要包括医疗照护与长期照护两大部分[④]。2015 年以前，在荷兰，长期照护从法律上是受到《特殊医疗费用支出法》（Exceptional Medical Expenses Act，EMEA，荷兰语简称 AWBZ）的保护。医疗照护涉及全科医生、专科医生、牙医、药剂师和治疗师提供的咨询、药物和治疗；另外，一些工具援助和运输也由医疗照护部门提供[⑤]。2015 年 1 月 1 日起，荷兰引入了《长期照护法》（Long-Term Care Act），从而取代了《特殊医疗费用支出法》，与《特殊医疗费用支出法》相比，新引入的《长期照护法》针对更加小范围的人群。其范围包括社会中最为脆弱的群体，例如晚期老年痴呆患者，严重身体或智力残疾患者等[⑥]。

---

① http：//countrymeters.info/en/Netherlands♯population_2017（2017-7-10）.
② The Netherlands Health system review. Health care translation，2010，12(1).
③ 史薇.荷兰老龄政策的经验与启示[J].老龄科学研究，2014，2(4)：70—79.
④ Rolden H J A，Rohling J H T，van Bodegom D，et al. Seasonal variation in Mortality，Medical care expenditure and institutionalization in older people：Evidence from a Dutch cohort of older health insurance clients [J]. PLOS One，2015，10(11)：1—14.
⑤ Schut E，Sorbe S Høj J. Health care reform and long-term care in the Netherlands [R]. OECD Economics Department Working Papers，2013，No. 1010.
⑥ Ministry of Public Health，Welfare and Sport. Healthcare in the Netherlands，https：//www. government. nl /documents /leaflets /2016 /02 /09 /healthcare-in-the-netherlands. (2018-1-8).

基本包裹包括①：医疗照护(包括全科医生的服务、医院、专科医生和产科医生)、住院、社区护理服务、初级和二级精神照护(包括心理医生和精神病治疗)、18 岁以前的心理治疗、18 岁以前的牙科治疗、各种医疗器械、各种处方药、产前护理、病人运送(包括急救)、辅助医疗、三段营养治疗周期、三段体外受精治疗周期、戒烟治疗、说话能力治疗。

1. 病人就诊流程

荷兰没有针对老年人的特殊医疗体系，在大多数情况下，所有年龄段的病人都需要首先与健康照护系统取得联系。病人的患病类型与严重程度决定了其就诊途径与提供方的类别(见案例1②)。

> **案例 1　一个需要膝关节置换术的女性患者**
>
> 首先，该患者需要联系签约的全科医生，全科医生根据其病情推荐相应的医院科室(本案例中为骨科)进行就诊。
>
> 该女性患者可以自由选择进入荷兰任何一家医院。她可以通过政府网站(www.kiesbeter.nl)对比医院的就诊等候时间及质量指标。等候时间在各个医院之间相差较大，从 2 周至 20 周不等。但只有少数患者会在网上进行对比，通常，患者会听从其全科医生的推荐或者选择最近的医院就诊。
>
> 接下来，由患者签约的全科医生或专科医生开具必要的药物。
>
> 转诊后，患者可能需要等候预约门诊医院专科医生的检查。
>
> 待专科医生检查完毕，该患者需要获得住院病人许可后才能进行手术。
>
> 在医院进行手术和初期康复之后，患者可选择回家，患者在家可能需要家庭照护(家庭护士和/或家庭助理)。对此，患者需要提出家庭照护评估申请。申请提交后由荷兰中央照护评估中心(荷兰语简称 CIZ：Centrum Indicatiestelling Zorg)对其进行评估。该申请由患者或者照护提供者提出均可。

---

① Healthcare. The medical system. https：//www. justlanded. com /english /Netherlands /Netherlands-Guide /Health /Healthcare. (2017-6-29).

② The Netherlands Health System review. Health care translation，2010，12(1).

2. 初级健康保健

荷兰初级保健采用的是全科医生守门人制度，这被认为是构成整个健康保健系统的强健基础。初级保健有效防止了使用不必要且更加昂贵的二级医疗。在荷兰，初级健康保健的提供者众多，有全科医生、物理治疗师、药剂师、心理学家、助产士等。[①]

3. 长期照护

长期照护包括机构与社区两大块。政府委托荷兰中央照护评估中心对长期照护开展评估，中心负责决定老年人是否需要长期照护，然后将评价结果发送给照护办公室。[①]

① **护理院和养老院照护（Residential Care）。** 2007 年，荷兰有 324 所护理院，960 所养老院和 210 所综合机构。2006 年，荷兰有 160 190 名老人居住在养老院或护理院，绝大多数是居住在养老院。护理院和养老院的区别在于医疗照护的提供程度有所不同。[①]

② **居家照护（Home Care）。** 居家照护服务由居家照护组织、养老院和护理院提供。在 80 岁以上的老人中，有 56% 的女性和 31% 的男性接受家庭照护。2007 年有 610 180 名老人接受不同类型的居家照护。数据显示，荷兰老年人接受居家照护的数量有稳步上升的趋势。[①]

（三）荷兰卫生体系改革

荷兰在历经近二十年的准备之后，于 2006 年开展了一轮大型卫生保健改革，此次改革为荷兰卫生体系带来了全新的管理机制和结构调整，引进了新的《健康保险法》（荷兰语简称 ZVW），并在 2007 年引入了《社会支持法》（荷兰语简称 WMO），WMO 的引进是为了取代《特殊医疗费用支出法》（AWBZ）的部分功能（比如提供家庭照护援助）。从 2013 年起，荷兰健康照护主要通过以上三项法案进行运作[②]。

这次改革中的一大亮点是荷兰政府的角色转变，即从以往直接控制卫生系统的角色转变为与卫生系统保持相应的距离并且不过多干预的角色。政府主要负责卫生保健的质量控制、可及性和可负担性，即创造一个公平、透明的环境，保障其卫生系统能顺利运行。因此，如今责任已经从政府转移到了保险

---

① The Nertherlands Health System review. Health care translation，2010，12（1）.
② 赵莹，郭林.荷德法三国医疗保障筹资改革[J]. 中国社会保障，2014（10）：36—37.

公司、提供方和病人[1][2]。

2006 年的改革引入了一项强制保险计划，即：健康保险公司可以在一定程度上与卫生保健提供方在照护的价格、体量和质量上进行协调，同时允许保险公司盈利并与股东分红。这意味着保险公司被赋予更多的权利。投保人也可以根据自己的需求自由选择保险公司和医疗服务提供者。这样的举措大大增加了保险公司之间的竞争，也刺激了医疗服务提供者在价格与服务质量方面的竞争，最终有利于控制医疗费用、提高医疗质量。但这种竞争并非完全市场化，而必须在政府的调控下进行有序竞争。自 2006 年 1 月 1 日起，每位荷兰公民都必须购买健康保险，否则将会被处以 130% 的年保险金作为罚金[3]。

针对长期照护，荷兰最近的一次大型改革是在 2015 年，此次改革的主要目的是控制支出增长，以维持长期照护的财政可持续性[4]。

（四）荷兰健康保健筹资及分配模式

荷兰的健康保险系统可以分为三大板块，即长期护理保险、基本医疗保险和自愿私人医疗保险[5][6]。其中，长期护理保险与后两种保险之间是互相平行又相互独立的系统，这三种保险一同为被保险人提供保障[1]。2013 年，荷兰健康保健的主要经费来自由强制保险（占支出总额的 72%，其中 43% 来自《健康保险法》ZVW，29% 来自长期护理《特殊医疗费用支出法》），13% 来源于政府，通过私人支出占总额的 13%，其中 9% 属于自费支付，4% 来源于补充性自愿性自愿保健保险 VHI），如图 6-9 所示。以下分别对三大板块进行介绍。

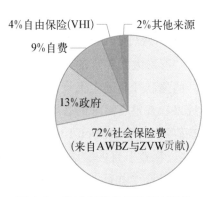

图 6-9　2015 年荷兰按经费来源的
卫生保健总支出百分比

来源：Statistics Netherlands 2015a.

---

① 　Rolden H. The Dutch health care system ［EB/OL］. Lyden Academy.

② 　Mot E，et al. The long-term care system for the elderly in the Netherlands. Netherlands：Enepri research report NO. 90 ［R］.2010，ISBN 978 9461380326.

③ 　赵莹，郭林.荷德法三国医疗保障筹资改革[J].中国社会保障，2014(10)：36—37.

④ 　Maarse，J. H.，&Jeurissen，P. P.(2016). The policy and politics of the 2015 long-term care reform in the Netherlands. Health Policy. 120(3)，241-245.

⑤ 　The Netherlands Health system review ［J］. Health care translation，2010，12 (1)：1—228.

⑥ 　Rolden H. The Dutch health care system ［EB/OL］. Lyden Academy.

　　第一大板块是长期护理保险，它受《特殊医疗费用支出法》保护，主要是为费用高昂的慢性病与持续照护提供保障，属于针对长期照护的强制社会健康保险计划（SHI）。特殊医疗费用支出法案主要规定了基于税收进行筹资的"政府保险"，所有荷兰公民均有义务每年缴纳他们应纳税额收入 12.15% 的费用（也包括 18 岁以下的公民和有工作的公民）。有意使用《特殊医疗费用支出法》照护的申请者需要经过荷兰中央照护评估中心的评估并获得其出具的照护需求证明，之后照护提供者方可向申请者提供相应的服务。该照护办公室独立运营，但与健康保险公司有密切联系。对于长期照护的提供者的费用，是通过对每一个病人的照护强度的评估来进行支付的。《特殊医疗费用支出法》由荷兰居民的税收办公室筹集的以收入为基准的定期缴款来提供资金。另外，接受长期照护的患者也需要分担支出，分担的总额取决于个体的收入，由中央监管办公室（CAK）进行征收。这两种资金来源都汇集到额外医疗支出总基金中（ATBZ），该基金由健康保健保险董事会（CVZ）进行管理①。

　　第二大板块是基本医疗保险，它受到《健康保险法》的保护，是覆盖全人群的强制社会健康保险计划（SHI）。基本健康保险覆盖有明确功效、具成本效果和有筹资需求的必要照护。荷兰基本卫生保险中的 59% 来自非政府财政筹资（Contribution-financed）。所有的经费来自两种方式：一是所谓的"名义保费"，直接缴纳给公民自主选择的保险公司；二是将保费从有收入的雇员工资中扣除，然后转到健康保健基金（Health Insurance Fund，HIF），HIF 用于补偿健康保险公司遇到的"不公平"，即保险公司可能会遇到高危客户，因此需要获得资金补偿以维持竞争力。HIF 的资金来源包括三个方面，45% 来自公民缴纳的费用，与雇员收入相关的缴纳金额占 50%，另外政府也向 HIF 出资（约占 5%）。2006 年的卫生改革主要就是针对这个板块。健康保险公司有权力与卫生保健提供者商议价格、体量和照护的质量，也允许盈利并与股东分红①。

　　第三大板块是自愿私人医疗保险，属于自由保险（VHI），这类保险不受《特殊医疗费用支出法》和《健康保险法》的制约，居民完全自愿购买①。

1. 社会支持法（WMO）

市政当局从国家政府的市政基金和市政税收中获得资金。每年，市政当

---

　　①　The Netherlands Health system review ［J］. Health care translation，2010，12（1）：1—228.

局都对《社会支持法》进行预算设定。通常，每个市政当局决定是否客户需要贡献资金，并给出计算方式。客户贡献资金通常用于上门照护服务、工具援助、住宅调整和个人预算①②。

2. 额外医疗支出法（特殊医疗费用支出法案）

在资金来源方面，保险基金由三部分构成，分别是：强制性保险费、合作付费和一般性税收补贴。强制性保险费占筹资来源的70%，凡年满15周岁并有纳税收入的公民都应缴纳与收入相关的保险费，15岁以下的儿童与15岁以上无纳税收入的公民不需要缴纳；合作付费占5%，这与受益者的收入存在相关性，收入水平是合作付费的重要考虑因素，收入水平低于一定标准的公民可以获得全部或部分减免；第三部分为一般性税收补贴。由于荷兰采取现收现付的财务模式，因此没有准备基金积累，即，如果当年的公共基金入不敷出，则会在来年提高保费以弥补亏损③。

3. 健康保险法（ZVW）

每一个18岁及以上的荷兰人均向健康保险公司缴纳名义保费（Nominal Fee）。不同的保险公司收费不同，但是政府设定了一个强制的免赔额。在2013年，免赔额为350欧元，但是居民可以选择将这个免赔额调整到最高850欧元，以此来降低他们的保险费用④。

2008年，名义保费平均为1 100欧元/年，约占2009年荷兰"模型收入"（由荷兰经济政策分析局定义，税前约为32 500欧元/年）净值的6%。2009年，名义保费从933欧元/年到1 150欧元/年不等。健康保险公司有自由设定名义保费水平的权利。被保险人直接向他们的保险公司支付保险费用。2015年，名义保费为1 158欧元/年。与收入相关的保费在2016年为年度应纳税额（最高限额为52 763欧元）的6.75%⑤。

（五）荷兰健康保健支付系统

荷兰长期照护保险制度没有规定给付上限，只对接受具体服务的需求量

①　Rolden H. The Dutch health care system［EB/OL］. Lyden Academy

②　Esther Mot et al. The long-term care system for the elderly in the Netherlands. Netherlands：Enepri research report NO. 90［R］. 2010，ISBN 978 9461380326.

③　方雨. 荷兰长期照护保险制度述评［J］. 中国医疗保险，2015（5）：68—70.

④　Rolden H. The Dutch health care system［EB/OL］. Lyden Academy.

⑤　MisjaMikkers R A. 2016. The Dutch healthcare system in international perspective.

进行了限制。被保险人可以根据需求选择接受实物给付或者现金给付，也可以选择将两种给付方式进行结合。

1. 居家照护

对居家照护的提供者提供的几乎所有类型的照护均按小时支付。群组的日间照护是特例。荷兰官方保健机构（The Dutch Healthcare Authority，NZA）决定《特殊医疗费用支出法》下的所有类型的照护的最高定价。例如，标准情况下，私人照护的最高定价为 42.96 欧元；特殊情况下是 64.94 欧元。区域照护办公室可以在最高定价下进行价格协商。根据《特殊医疗费用支出法》，接受长期照护的人需要满足以下条件：由于身体、老年心理疾病或精神疾病或精神、身体或感官障碍导致无法对其提供基本照护的人[①]。

2. 机构照护

如今，每一个机构照护的潜在使用者在接受评估以后，评估方会根据使用者的特定需求给出一个照护组合决定。对于每一个组合，NZA 都有一个固定的价格表，该价格不允许协商。服务组合是按天支付，对于护理和照护的价格从 56.44 欧元（不包括治疗）到 216.92 欧元（包括治疗）。原则上，从服务使用者选择机构那一天开始，该机构就开始收到按天支付的费用，直到使用者选择另一家机构为止[②]。

（六）荷兰老龄人口健康服务的模式和特点

与其他 OECD 国家一样，荷兰也面临着如何以一种具有成本效益的方式为老龄化人群提供高质量卫生和长期照护服务的挑战。

1. 长期照护

从 1968 年起，荷兰就已经建立起了长期照护保险系统。长期照护保险系统是荷兰健康保健系统的重要组成部分，占其健康照护预算的 38%。每一个居住在荷兰的公民都受到《特殊医疗费用支出法》的保护，该法案不仅包含老年照护，也包括所有慢性病照护，尤其关注私人保险市场无法覆盖的且花费高昂的慢性病的照护。目前，该法案覆盖了居家和机构老年照护、机构中针对精

---

① Schut E, Sorbe S, Høj J. Health care reform and long-term care in the Netherlands [R]. OECD Economics Department Working Papers, 2013, No. 1010.

② 方雨.荷兰长期照护保险制度述评[J].中国医疗保险,2015 (5)：68—70.

神和身体残疾的照护以及慢性精神病人的机构照护。

特殊医疗费用支出法案服务的覆盖范围较广，包括私人照护、护理、援助、机构中的治疗。援助包括以一对多的日间照护和私人援助（一对一）。援助的目的是让老人尽可能保持独立的能力（如帮助组织或管理家庭）。在过去，这样的支持意在改善社会参与（如散步、去商店或教堂、外出）。荷兰政府努力使《特殊医疗费用支出法》的支出处于预算之内。每一届政府换届之后都会对荷兰未来四年《特殊医疗费用支出法》的支出做出新的规划，而规划是基于新政府政策和长期照护的预期需求[①]。

《特殊医疗费用支出法》是国家针对长期照护而制定的保险计划，主要针对院内照护。它主要在六大方面提供资金帮助：（a）私人照护：帮助洗澡、穿衣、刮胡子、上洗手间等；（b）护理：包括伤口清洗、注射、自我照护的教学等；（c）咨询：帮助组织日常练习事宜，如煮咖啡或填表；（d）治疗：帮助从疾病或伤害中恢复（如，中风后学习如何走路）或改善行为或生活技巧；（e）长期居住在养老院或护理院；（f）特定机构的短期居住（一周最多三个全天）。

2. 需求评估

由于 2006 年的改革，卫生保健提供者的支付方式也发生了彻底的转变。如今，家庭医生通过人头税和按项目付费的混合方式获得薪资。长期照护提供者是通过照护强化包裹获得薪资的。每一个患者的照护强度都需要经过独立评估。[②]

每一个《特殊医疗费用支出法》照护请求都需要经过独立评估机构 CIZ 的评估。CIZ 在评估上不存在经济利益，它的评估决定不会影响其机构的经济地位。因此，评估是独立、客观和整合的评估。申请者仅在满足如下一个或多个因素时才有资格接受特殊医疗费用支出法案照护：（a）躯体的、老年病的精神或精神紊乱或受限；（b）智力的、身体感觉的残疾。CIZ 采用一套特定的标准来判定一个人是否有资格获得一项或多项《特殊医疗费用支出法》照护服务：协助、私人照护、护理、机构治疗、精神病原因导致的延期滞留。对于每项服务，其必要照护的总量需要经过测量而确定。[③]

---

① Bettio F，Verashchagina A. Long-term care for the elderly. Provisions and providers in 33 European countries. Rome：Fondazione G，Brodolini，2010.

② The Netherlands Health system review. Health care translation，2010，12(1)

③ Esther Mot et al. The long-term care system for the elderly in the Netherlands. Netherlands：ENEPRI research report NO. 90 ［R］. 2010，ISBN 978 9461380326.

　　CIZ 采用一个称之为漏斗型的评估模型（见图 6-10）。第一步，CIZ 分析特殊医疗费用支出法案潜在收益者的情况。它不仅仅考虑到紊乱和功能受限，也考虑到该申请人在何种环境下使用什么样的功能。第二步，CIZ 决定怎样更好地解决潜在客户的照护问题。在决定提供《特殊医疗费用支出法》照护服务之前，CIZ 考虑三个方面的解决办法：一是接受普通照护（必要的时候由家庭成员提供喘息照护）；二是使用其他公共资金覆盖的供给，这些供给先于特殊医疗费用支出法案照护的使用；三是使用人人可以获得的普通供给，比如家庭购物快递服务、幼儿照护等。第二步的结果是根据照护的种类、体量、评估的有效性的时期与交付条件来决定《特殊医疗费用支出法》照护（包括家庭成员的普通照护）的总需求。第三步关注的是志愿照护可能扮演的角色。家庭成员理应提供普通照护，但是除此以外的任何帮助都属于志愿服务。这意味着非正式照护超出了普通照护。被保险者可以申请私人预算用于支付非正式照护。评估决定中可以包括一定形式的喘息照护，以此来支持非正式照护的照护提供者。第四步，CIZ 做出在机构或在家接受照护的决定。①

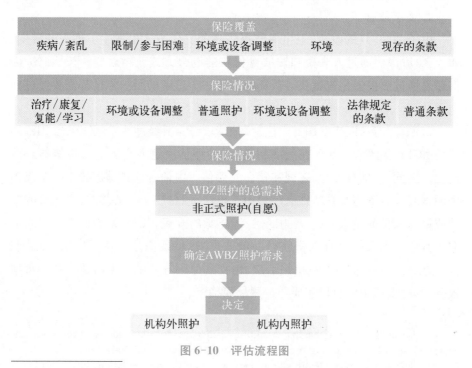

图 6-10　评估流程图

　　①　Esther Mot et al. The long-term care system for the elderly in the Netherlands. Netherlands：ENEPRI research report NO. 90 ［R］. 2010，ISBN 978 9461380326.

（七）发展愿景

与欧洲其他国家相比，荷兰老年人接受专业照护的比例相对较高，约 18% 的 65 岁及以上的老人接受家庭照护①②。但在 2015 年，荷兰进行了以"去机构化"为目的的长期护理和养老体系的改革，旨在让更多的老人重新回到以居家养老为主要模式的养老体系中去。此次改革使得荷兰老年公寓和养老院养老人口数量锐减，从改革前的 80 万下降到改革后的 20 万。与此同时，中央政府的护理和养老事务管理权也更多地下放到了当地政府和医保公司③。荷兰政府对于长期照护有两个比较宏观的目标：一是关注居民自身的责任和其周围的网络，如朋友、家人和邻居，而不是像往常一样关注正式照护系统；二是明确区分个体责任、健康照护的权利与实际解决方法。荷兰当局希望在未来（十年或更长时间）彻底废除《特殊医疗费用支出法》体系。这个长期目标将分步完成。首先，私人照护、咨询、日常活动和其他目前通过《特殊医疗费用支出法》提供的服务都应该通过《社会支持法》WMO 来提供。因为这些活动与社会支持更相关，更有可能通过病人的社会网络进行提供，因此当地市政当局或许能比国家的《特殊医疗费用支出法》体系更好地提供这些服务。其次，安排短期和长期居住和设备使用是客户自己的责任，不再由公共资源提供。最后，照护应该由《健康保险法》提供，因为它更多地涉及医疗照护而不是长期照护或者社会支持。④

2013 年 9 月 9 日，荷兰卫生、福利和体育部部长 Schippers 女士在北京举办的中荷卫生研讨会上表示："初级卫生保健将成为未来医疗的主力。在未来，荷兰全科医生基层医疗守门人的角色将进一步加强，他们将被赋予更多的责任。患者所有不太复杂的疾病都将更多地交给全科医生来解决。"

（八）启示

不同的国家根据其国情选择不同的健康保健体系，如英国和丹麦等国家

---

① Bettio，F.，& Verashchagina，A. Long-term care for the elderly. Provisions and providers in 33 European countries. Rome：Fondazione G，Brodolini，2010.

② Allen K，Bednarik R，Campbell L，et al. Governance and finance of long-term care across Europe，Overview Paper［R］. United Kingdom/Vienna：University of Birmingham/European Centre for Social Welfare Policy and Research：Birmingham，2011.

③ 荷兰养老欧洲第一的秘密：提倡健康衰老，鼓励老人做完整的人［EB/OL］. http：//www.thepaper.cn/newsDetail_forward_1565324（2017-12-19）.

④ Misja Mikkers RA. 2016. The Dutch healthcare system in international perspective.

在健康保健的保险和提供方面都涉及，然而有些国家则只是针对特定的人群才作为保险方的角色进行服务，如美国针对老年人的 Medicare，针对穷人的 Medicaid 和针对退伍军人的 Veterans Affairs①。

1. 没有完美的健康保健体系

然而，每一种体系都会存在其缺点，即便是发达国家也是如此。通过欧洲健康消费指数（EHCI）2006—2015 年的报告分析可以看出，排名靠前的国家均为采用俾斯麦（Bismarck②）体系的国家和采用贝弗里奇③的人口稀少的国家（如瑞典等北欧国家）。而人口较多的采用贝弗里奇体系的国家似乎很难在消费价值方面取得优异的表现，如最大的贝弗里奇国家英国、西班牙和意大利。荷兰的竞争型健康保健模式在本国也存在争议，反对者认为"竞争会鼓励供给、增加需求和支出，从而导致健康保健变成盈利的部门"，认为"竞争是一个灾难，健康保健不应该是一个市场"，然而，支持者则认为"竞争最终让健康保健部门提供符合客户需求的健康服务。竞争会让我们摆脱在等候名单上耗费时间，也会让质量和供给更加出色。因此竞争是幸事而不应该成为烦恼"④。

2. 发扬居家养老

和西方国家相比，我国有着历史悠久的家庭养老传统（非正式照护），子女、亲属在养老方面扮演着重要的角色。虽然当代社会由于人口迁徙等原因引起了家庭养老功能的弱化，但作为有着该养老传统与意识的国家，我们应当意识到自身优势。上海作为全国拥有老年人比例最高的国际大都市，应该在借鉴发达国家健康保健体系的基础上，根据其特点进行针对性的健康体系设计，荷兰特有的"政府调控下的市场主导型"有其可取之处，尤其是其特有的三方（个体、保险提供方、保健提供方）相互制衡的模式值得思考，但并非完全适合我国现有国情，因为荷兰整个国家的医疗水平相对均衡，而我国则存在医疗水平及资源差异化等问题。因此，建议在决定依靠市场相互制衡之前进行充分的论证与全方位的考虑，以探索出一条适合我国文化传统和社会经济状况的老龄化应对方式。

---

①　Misja Mikkers RA. 2016. The Dutch healthcare system in international perspective.

②　俾斯麦健康体系：基于社会保险，有多方保险机构参与，与健康保健提供者在组织上相互独立。

③　贝弗里奇健康体系：资金和服务提供均在一个组织体系内。如英国的 NHS。

④　de Vries M，Kossen J. How does the healthcare market operate? This is how Dutch healthcare works［M］. Netherlands：De Argumentenfabriek，2015.

四、德国应对老龄化健康保障的经验及启示

(一) 德国老龄化的进程及其伴随的问题

德国早在 20 世纪 50 年代就步入了老龄化社会,目前已经成为世界上人口老龄化程度最严重的国家之一。根据德国联邦统计局的最新数据,2013 年,德国 65 岁及以上人口至少占总人口的 21%,75 岁及以上人口是新生儿的 2 倍,80 岁以上人口占总人口的 5.4%。预计到 2060 年,德国 65 岁及以上人口将至少达到总人口的 1/3,80 岁及以上人口将达到总人口的 13%[①]。由于人体在衰老的过程中身体机能逐步受损、衰退,老年人的疾病风险与伤害发生率会更高。2013 年,德国对各年龄段人口健康状况的统计分析数据显示[②],60~65 岁、70~75 岁、75 岁以上老年人口的疾病与伤害发生率分别为17.6%、21.1%、28.2%,远高于社会青壮年(见图 6-11)。因此,人口的老龄化必然会给社会的健康乃至经济带来一定的压力。

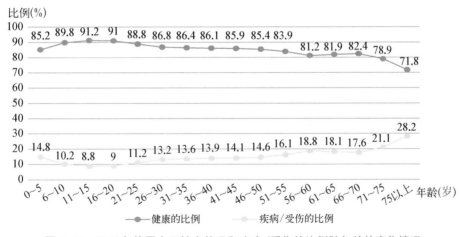

图 6-11 2013 年德国人口健康状况和疾病/受伤的比例随年龄的变化情况

① Federal Statistical Office of Germany. German's population by 2060:Results of the 13th coordinated population projection [EB/OL]. https://www.destatis.de/EN/Publications/Specialized/Population/Population.html.

② Federal Statistical Office of Germany. Sick and injured people by age-group and sex [EB/OL]. https://www.destatis.de/EN/FactsFigures/SocietyState/Health/HealthStatusBehaviourRelevantHealth/Tables/SickAndInjuredPeople.html.

　　人口老龄化的负担在德国医疗卫生费用的分布上体现非常明显。2010年，德国人均医疗卫生费用为2 421欧元，66～70岁、71～75岁老年人的平均医疗费用分别为总人口平均医疗费用的147%、174%，76～80岁、81～85岁、86～90岁老年人的平均医疗费用分为总人口平均医疗费用的210%、234%、248%，而1～25岁人口的医疗费用均在人均医疗卫生费用的50%以下（见图6-12）①。随着年龄的增长，人均医疗费上涨明显，人口老龄化带来的社会问题由此可见一斑。

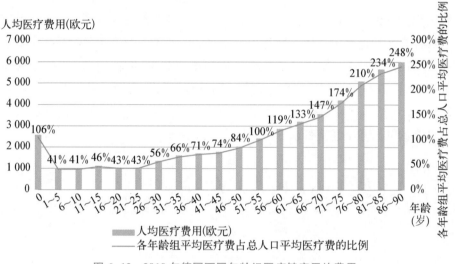

图6-12　2010年德国不同年龄组医疗健康平均费用

（二）德国老年人的健康保障状况

　　德国是一个社会保险型国家，通过基于收入的保费筹集和基于需要的保费支出实现社会不同群体之间的风险共担、团结互助。德国的健康保险由医疗保险和护理保险两大部分组成，健康服务也相应分为医疗服务和护理服务两个部分。医疗卫生费用主要来自保险筹资，医疗保险为主，其他保险为辅。2012年德国的卫生总费用中，法定医疗保险支付占57%，私人医疗保险支付占9%，长期护理保险、事故保险、养老保险支付分别占8%、2%、1%。此外还有一部分费用来自个人、社会团体、企业和国家，其中个人自付（或非政府组织

---

①　隋学礼.德国医保筹资制度的改革路径分析——基于人口老龄化和家庭政策视角[J].北京航空航天大学学报（社会科学版），2016（2）：13—19.

资助)部分占 14%,国家税收支付占 5%,雇主支付占 4%[①]。

1.医疗保障体系

德国医疗保险由法定医疗保险和私人医疗保险两大运行系统构成。按照德国的法律,根据雇员的收入标准来确定参加医疗保险的类型,低收入者必须参加法定医疗保险,而高收入者可以自由选择法定医疗保险或私人医疗保险。除此之外,还有两类群体不需要参加法定医疗保险,一类是国家公务员,一类是自我雇佣人员(包括企业家),前者必须购买私人医疗保险,后者可以选择购买私人医疗保险或者完全自理[②]。法定医疗保险是德国医疗保障体系的主要组成部分,由国内 154 家非营利性的疾病基金运行。私人医疗保险对某些职业群体来说是强制性的,如公务员;对其他人来说则是在法定医疗保险之外的备选方案,一部分参加法定医疗保险的人,如收入超过一定阈值的自雇主和雇员,会再选择买一份私人保险为自己提供补充保障。根据 2013 年的数据,法定医疗保险覆盖了德国 85% 的公民,其中强制性成员占 35%,其家属占18%;退休人员占 21%,其家属占 2%;自愿参加者占 5%,其家属占 4%。私人医疗保险覆盖了德国约 11% 的公民(其中个体经营者和国家公务员是最大的购买群体),其中公务员及其家属大约占 5%(包括退休的公务员以及依靠他们的受扶养人)。特殊人群医疗保险覆盖了剩余 4% 的人群,包括军人、警察等。

法定医疗保险缴费由雇主和雇员按照 1∶1 的比例共同负担,缴费多少取决于收入而不取决于风险。根据"家庭免费联动保险原则"[③],雇员的子女及其低收入配偶跟在其名下,无需缴费即为法定医疗保险所覆盖。退休人员和失业人员分别由养老人与残疾人保险法定计划的机构和联邦就业机构为其承担雇主的缴费融资角色,为他们缴纳医疗保费中由原雇主承担的部分。

医疗服务的提供者为医院与门诊,作为医疗服务享用者的患者并不直接向医疗服务提供者直接付费,而是由疾病基金向医疗服务提供者间接付费。患者就诊仅负担少量自付费用,一般来说患者自付(OOP)费用最多不能超过其家庭收入的 2%,对于一些严重的慢性病患者,自付费用最多不能超过其家

---

① Busse R,Blümel M. Germany:Health system review [J]. Health Systems in Transition,2014,16(2):1—296.

② 李乐乐,张知新,王辰.德国医疗保险制度对我国统筹发展的借鉴与思考[J].中国医院管理,2016,36(11):94—96.

③ 陈翔,王小丽.德国社会医疗保险筹资、支付机制及其启示[J].卫生经济研究,2009(12):20—22.

庭收入的 1%①。2011 年,这种自付的比例占医疗总支出的 13.2%,主要涵盖医药、养老服务和医疗救助等领域②。德国的住院费用支付目前全部采用 DRGs 付费,费用支付标准每年由住院医师协会(或医院)和保险公司协商签订协议确定。

2. 护理保障体系

1990 年,统一后的德国人口自然增长率为零。到 1995 年,德国 60 岁以上的老龄人口占比已高达 21%。人口的快速老龄化使德国的长期护理需求急剧膨胀。但是德国缺乏一套完整的护理服务提供体系和资金保障机制,老年人的护理费用由个人负担,个人无法负担时,则需要依靠社会救助,70%入住机构的老年人需要通过社会救助支付护理费。由于社会救助费用由州和自治体负担,导致州和自治体的财政负担过重③。在这样的背景下,1994 年,德国颁布了《护理保险法》,并于 1995 年 1 月 1 日开始逐步实施④,确保老年人能够享有必要的护理服务,同时减轻政府的财政负担。据德国联邦统计局提供的数字,2006 年,参加法定及私人护理保险者已分别达 7 137 万人和 848 万人,享受护理者达 181 万余人,其中 2/3 是 75 岁以上的老年人。

德国现行的护理保险体系实行"护理保险跟随医疗保险"原则,即所有参加医疗保险的人都要参加护理保险,其中参加法定医疗保险者加入法定护理保险,参加私人医疗保险者加入私人护理保险⑤。护理保险费与医疗保险费一同征收,由雇主和雇员按收入的一定比例缴纳。从 2017 年起,护理保险费率为收入的 2.55%,雇主和雇员各承担一半。对于退休人员,保费需要自己完全负担;对于失业者、领取救助金的难民等,保费由政府负担;对于无子女者,考虑到他们将来无法得到来自家庭的非正式照顾,费率加收 0.25%⑥。护理保险采用现收现付的财务模式,现收保费用于当期,遵循社会互助与个人自助相结

---

①　马里恩·卡斯佩斯—梅尔克.德国的卫生体制——特点、问题与解决方案[J].社会保障研究,2006(2):106—112.

②　刘权,邓勇.德国医疗卫生体制的新变与启示[J].中国医院院长,2016(15):66—71.

③　于建明.德国的长期护理服务体系及启示[J].中国民政,2017(3):57—58.

④　刘源,赵晶晶.德国的医疗保险和护理保险[J].保险研究,2008(3):89—91.

⑤　郝丽燕,杨士林.德国社会护理保险制度的困境与未来发展方向[J].德国研究,2015(2):100—113.

⑥　王敏,李彦,孙晓阳.长期护理保险筹资机制研究——以德国和日本经验为例[J].医学与法学,2017,9(1):49—54.

合、收支定价制与风险定价制相结合的原则。

保险给付时,受益人可以选择机构护理也可以选择家庭护理,可以选择实物给付也可以选择现金给付,其中实物给付是指由专业的服务提供者为需求者提供个人卫生、营养摄取、行动和家务上的帮助。但是德国的长期护理保险为部分保险,采用成本分担机制,每种形式的护理服务都有封顶给付标准(见表 6-5),护理级别越高受益金额越高,对于超出部分,受益人要用自己的收入或财产进行补充[①]。对于选择家庭护理的,他们没有需要缴纳的护理费用共付部分,但是当每个月护理费用超出护理基金给付的额度时,受益人需自行负担或申请社会救助[②];对于选择机构护理的,他们需要自付食宿费用,以及至少 25% 的护理费用。一些研究显示,机构护理中受益人实际自付比例接近 50%。此外,对于需要耐用性的医疗装置或其他技术性辅助设备(如床或轮椅)、消耗性产品、家庭改造的受益人,也需要自付一部分费用[③]。

表 6-5　德国家庭护理和机构护理的月给付标准

服务/给付形式		Ⅰ级护理	Ⅱ级护理	Ⅲ级护理	特别个案护理	
居家护理	实物给付	450 欧	1 100 欧	1 550 欧	—	
	照护津贴	235 欧	440 欧	700 欧	—	
日间护理或夜间护理		450 欧	1 100 欧	1 550 欧	—	
完全机构护理		1 023 欧	1 279 欧	1 550 欧	1 918 欧	

(三) 德国老年人的健康服务提供状况

1. 医疗服务提供

德国健康服务体系按功能大致划分为四类,各自的业务范围和分工比较明确。一是私人诊所,由开业医生自己筹资建立,大部分为全科医生,主要负责一般门诊检查、咨询等,通过提供医疗服务获得收入。私人诊所不提供住院

---

① 郝君富,李心愉.德国长期护理保险:制度设计、经济影响与启示[J].人口学刊,2014(2):104—112.

② 陈雷.德国养老长期照护政策:目标、资金及给付服务内涵[J].中国民政,2016,(17):36—37.

③ Gibson,M J. Redfoot,D L. Comparing long-term care[EB/OL]. https://assets.aarp.org/rgcenter/il/2007_19_usgerman_ltc.pdf.

服务,但允许借用医院的手术室和设备实施适宜的手术。二是医院,主要负责提供各种形式的住院治疗服务,除急诊外,不提供门诊服务,教学医院因研究和教学目的才设有门诊。每个区域都有明确的医院规划,按标准设置四级医疗机构。区域内医院的等级和规模、设备条件、功能由政府根据服务的需要统一安排划定,不同级别的医院提供不同层服务①。三是康复机构,主要负责病人出院治疗后的康复工作。四是护理机构,主要负责老年人以及残疾人士的护理工作。康复和护理机构以公立和非营利医院为主②。

每一个参加保险的人,都可以自由选择一位开业医生提供基本诊疗服务,并且可以转换。个人选择医生后,开业医生要为其建立专门健康档案。发生疾病时,可以自由选择到诊所、医院以及康复机构等进行就诊③。但是由于综合医院并不承担门诊医疗任务,大量的门诊患者必须首先到全科诊所或专科诊所就诊。如有必要,再由全科医生转诊到专科医院或综合医院。同时,医疗保险公司作为医疗服务的付费方,如果发现医院接诊"小病"患者,则费用全部由医院承担,保险公司不予支付。同样,一旦发现诊所将"小病"转诊到大医院,保险公司也会对诊所采取诸如降低支付比例或扣款等严厉措施。严格的分级体系与第三方支付机制,为德国的医疗秩序提供了保障④。如果参保人员承诺年度内门诊只在某个医师处就诊,法定保险机构将给予该参保人员额外的优惠,如提供健康体检和一些健身器材等,以鼓励参保人员利用费用低的门诊服务。

德国的医疗服务体系基本分为门诊和住院两个体系,分工明确,但是合作不足。不过,德国的医疗服务体系也在不断进行着改革和创新。在最近几年的改革中,德国政府逐步将门急诊服务和住院服务进行合作,如允许部分开业医师利用医院手术室,允许部分医院工作人员在业余时间看门急诊,近年来又开始探索健康服务整合提供模式,开展疾病管理计划,这些举措在提高老年人医疗服务的可及性方面起到重要的作用,门急诊是德国医疗服务体系应对老龄化的特色与经验。

---

① 余红星,冯友梅,付旻,等.医疗机构分工协作的国际经验及启示——基于英国、德国、新加坡和美国的分析[J].中国卫生政策研究,2014(6):10—15.
② 李滔,张帆.德国医疗卫生体制改革现状与启示[J].中国卫生经济,2015(4):92—96.
③ 王丙毅,尹音频.德国医疗管制模式的特点、改革取向及借鉴意义[J].理论学刊,2008(7):58—61.
④ 魏鹏.德国分级医疗体系管窥[J].中国医疗保险,2011(9):70.

人口老龄化与疾病谱的变化促使德国不断进行健康服务整合探索。从1993年开始,德国法律就允许跨部门的医疗服务试点项目,为疾病基金协会与健康服务提供者创造了尝试整合服务模式的机会。2000年,整合服务合约引入医疗卫生服务体系,通过推动急诊部门与住院部门、专科医生与全科医生、医疗服务提供者与非医疗服务提供者(如普通护理服务提供者)、预防中心与康复中心之间的密切合作,来实现跨部门的、以病人为中心的、多学科交叉的健康服务提供模式。整合服务基于整合服务合约,只要求各服务提供方同意,因此实际操作中有很多不同的服务整合项目。比如,德国的巴伐利亚州有健康区域建设项目、德国北部西波美拉尼亚地区应对老年人的医疗需求建立了痴呆照顾整合模式。

疾病管理计划是一项对针对慢性病患者的医疗服务进行改进的计划。同时,它也是德国医疗服务结构进行整合的一种尝试,它将某个特定疾病群体整个病程所需的健康服务组织起来,协调、改进服务提供者之间的互动,使服务的提供能够与需求更一致、更有效。根据德国联邦委员会的规定,纳入慢病管理计划的疾病必须具备以下条件:(a)患病率高;(b)疾病治疗费用高;(c)现有疾病管理措施能有效提高患者健康水平;(d)能建立科学的临床循证指南;(e)管理服务开展需多部门合作;(f)自我管理对健康结果影响较大。目前,德国纳入疾病管理计划的病种包括糖尿病、心脏病、心功能不全、哮喘、乳腺癌、慢性阻塞性肺疾病六种。慢性病管理计划由患者自愿选择是否参加。患者在注册加入慢性病管理计划前必须选择一位参与其慢性病管理的初级保健医生(通常是患者的家庭医生)作为慢性病管理协调医师。协调医师对患者的慢性病进行确诊,然后根据风险结构补偿计划管理条例将符合条件的慢性病患者纳入慢性病管理计划,并为其制定慢性病管理计划。此外,协调医师负责向慢性病患者提供咨询服务,就治疗目标与慢性病注册患者达成共识,对患者进行健康教育,协调安排治疗项目,遵循临床循证指南开展慢性病管理相关服务,并完成慢性病管理计划协议中涉及的质量目标及疾病管理文件记录工作等。必要时,协调医师需要将注册患者向专科医院或综合医院进行转诊。一般来说,专科医院主要负责慢性病并发症以及合并症的治疗、年度健康体检及计划怀孕等,综合医院主要负责注册患者的急诊服务。慢性病管理服务由地方保险基金分别对协调医师与医院通过按人头付费和按服务项目付费的方式进行支付,同时地方社会保险负责制定服务提供者(协调医师)的准入条件并对其服务质量进行审核监管①。

2. 老年护理服务提供

因老年人身体或精神方面的问题，老年护理服务需要在较长一段时间内（至少 6 个月以上），在包括卫生、饮食、行动、家务四个方面的日常生活行为中，至少有两个方面经常性或实质性地帮助老年人。同时被保险的老年人必须通过申请，经过医疗审查委员会的评定才能成为护理对象，评估组成员主要由在老年医学方面受过训练的护士和医生组成，他们通过观察申请人所处的家庭及社会环境，运用国家标准量表对申请人的健康与功能状况进行评估，得出申请人护理需求评定结果。

护理需求划分主要取决于老年人所需要的护理时间和护理频率。一级护理每天至少需要一次、至少 90 分钟的日常生活护理服务；二级护理每天至少需要三次、至少 3 个小时的日常生活护理服务；三级护理是最高级别的护理，需要一天 24 小时不定次数、至少 5 个小时的日常生活护理服务。德国的长期护理保险在给付形式上给了老年人一定的自由权，他们可以选择护理服务的给付形式（现金或实物）以及护理服务的提供场所（居家或机构）。但是在制度设计上仍然体现着"居家护理先于机构护理"的原则，通过向家庭护理提供者提供护理津贴、假期、社会保险等方式，鼓励居家护理并由家属提供服务。

（四）德国应对老龄化健康保障问题的经验

1. 完善的服务提供体系是老年人健康保障的基础

作为一个保险型福利国家，社会保险责任共担、团结互助的内涵在德国的医疗保险中得到了充分体现。医疗保险缴费的标准只与收入相关，与风险无关，疾病风险在不同年龄段、不同职业的人群中间调节均衡。在制度建设上，我国与德国极为相似。但是，德国的医疗服务提供的整合模式与疾病管理计划的开展，是提高老年人医疗服务的可及性、化解老龄化压力的可行路径。近两年，社区的健康管理、整合服务在我国也受到越来越多的关注，在探索的过程中，我国可以借鉴德国经验。

2. 老年护理保障制度是老年人健康保障的重要部分

为了满足老龄化带来的护理需求，德国建立了专门的护理保险制度，旨在使有护理需求的老年人在需要护理服务时有一定的经济保障。从实施效果来

---

① 周建再，代宝珍.德国慢性病管理现状[J].中国社会保障,2016(12)：75—77.

看,一方面是长期护理保险确实使老年人从中受益,使他们在基本护理服务的获得上有了一定的保障;另一方面,长期护理保险的引入使德国的社会救助支出在两年内节省了接近 60%①,也使医疗卫生支出中依靠税收筹集的比重从1996 年的 10.8%下降到 2012 年的 4.8%,这样使政府的财政压力得到很好的缓解。

我国自 1999 年步入老龄化社会,老龄化的程度在不断加深,到 2015 年,我国 65 岁及以上人口已经达到 1.44 亿人,占总人口的 10.5%。随着经济社会发展、传统观念改变以及家庭结构变迁,我国的空巢老人、留守老人越来越多,我国老年人长期照顾问题既成为一种社会需求,也成为一种社会风险。借鉴德国的经验,我国应该结合国情,考虑护理保险的建立实施,进一步完善对老年人的健康保障。

---

① 施巍巍,刘一姣. 德国长期照护保险制度研究及其启示[J]. 商业研究,2011(3):98—105.

第七章

应对老龄化挑战的十大策略

【导读】

应对人口老龄化是全社会的共同责任,也是一项涉及多领域、多层面的系统工程。积极开展应对人口老龄化的行动,关键在于制定、实施有效的公共政策和其他相关配套政策。本章从优化筹资、转变服务模式、统筹资源配置、合理控费、促进公平、应用信息化等方面出发,提出应对老龄化挑战的十大策略,旨在形成一股维护、促进健康老龄化的强大合力,为中央及地方政府积极应对老龄化挑战提供思路和借鉴。

一、应对老龄化：迎接筹资挑战

卫生筹资政策应与老年人全民健康覆盖最终目标相一致，即确保所有人都能获取所需的卫生服务，如疾病预防、健康促进、疾病处置和康复治疗等，且在获取卫生服务时没有经济障碍①。据上海市社会科学院预测②，上海市常住人口总量将呈持续增长态势，2020 年预计人口总量达 2 650.1 万人，持续增长到 2035 年（2 871.5 万人）后开始回落，2050 年预计达到 2 778.3 万人。与此同时，老龄化趋势不断加深，预计到 2020 年 60 岁及以上老年人占比达到 21.5%，2050 年达到44.8%。与之相对应，本研究结合 2010—2015 年人均卫生总费用变化趋势，利用指数回归模型预测医疗费用，预测全市常住人口医疗费用将逐年上涨，由 2015 年的 1 072.0 亿元上升到 2020 年的 1 861.8 亿元，2050 年预计达到 8 841.5 亿元，其中，60 岁及以上老年人医疗费用占比将由 2015 年的 54.4% 上升到 2020 年的58.0%，2050 年占比预计达到 80.8%。近年来，上海市经济增长放缓，GDP 增长率由 2011 年的 8.2% 下降到 2016 年的 6.8%；一般性公共预算收入增长率也由2011 年的 19.4% 下降到 2016 年的 16.1%。从筹资结构来看，上海市卫生总费用以社会卫生支出为主，占比近 60%，在全国处于最高水平。政府卫生支出占比则略高于 20%，近年来政府卫生支出占财政支出的比例也略有下降，由 2011 年的5.5% 下降到 2015 年的 5.2%。针对老龄化带来的巨额医疗费用增长，亟须构建一个结构合理、可持续发展的筹资体系。

（一）拓展筹资渠道，优化筹资结构

目前，上海市针对老年人群的医疗保障制度在结构上相对割裂，碎片化的保障体系导致不同社会群体保障待遇差别显著，保障公平性受损，保障制度管

---

① World health report 2010. Health systems financing: the path to universal coverage [EB/OL].Geneva: World Health Organization, 2010. http://www.who.int/whr/2010/en/.

② 周海旺.上海人口老龄化趋势与完善养老服务模式研究[J]. 上海金融学院学报，2011(4)：37—49.

理效果不佳。建议通过顶层设计，明确基本医保的保障范围和政府卫生支出责任，拓展筹资渠道，构建符合上海市实际情况的、以社会保险为基础、商业保险为补充、社会救济和社会福利托底的健康老龄化保障体系，对居家、社区、机构的保障政策进行整合统一。

一是拓宽多元化医保筹资渠道。不同年龄、不同经济水平的人群对医疗服务的需求不同，虽然上海市常住人口基本实现医保全覆盖，但各保障制度间医疗费用负担存在较大差异，结合医保人群和基金运行情况来看，居民医保和新农合保障人群中老年人比例高，职工医保个人账户基金结余多集中在年轻人群。目前商业医疗保险市场上针对老年人的险种少、市场小，可探索将基本医保和商业医保相结合，共同发展，如完善职工医保个人账户功能，鼓励购买商业健康保险等。2016年12月，上海市人民政府印发《关于职工自愿使用医保个人账户历年结余资金购买商业保险有关事项的通知》（沪府发〔2016〕106号），其中明确规定，上海市职工基本医疗保险参保人员，可以按照自愿原则使用职工医保个人账户历年结余资金，为本人购买经中国保险监督管理委员会批准的、上海市政府同意的商业医疗保险专属产品。上海保险业针对此项政策开发了两款低保费、高保障的专属商业保险产品：一款是住院自费费用保险产品，为全国首款覆盖老年人群的住院自费费用个人健康保险产品，对合理且必要的自费医疗费用，按50%的比例进行赔付；另一款是改进型重大疾病产品，在扩展市场上现有产品保障病种范围的基础上，保费大幅低于市场同类产品价格①。该项政策的推行使得多方得益：从政府角度看，有助于城镇职工基本医保制度持续稳定发展，提高个人账户资金使用效率；从保险行业角度看，有助于进一步扩大商业保险覆盖面，更好地发挥其在多层次医疗保障体系中的作用；从受保障人群看，有助于减轻医保外自费费用负担和重大疾病医疗费用负担，有效化解城镇职工因病致贫、因病返贫的风险。

二是发展长期护理保险。随着老龄化程度加深，老年人的护理需求日益增多，护理服务负担也逐步加大。建立长期护理保险，有利于保障失能人员基本生活权益，提升生活质量，使其生活更为体面且富有尊严，有利于弘扬中国传统文化，有利于增进人民福祉，促进社会公平正义，维护社会稳定。2016年12月，上海市人民政府印发《上海市长期护理保险试点办法》（沪府发〔2016

---

① 上海：明年起职工医保个人账户可购买商业保险.http：//business.sohu.com/20161227/n477100888.shtml.

110 号),两年试点期内针对 60 周岁及以上、经评估失能程度达到评估等级二至六级且在评估有效期内的参保人员提供长期护理保险待遇,包括社区居家照护、养老机构照护和住院医疗护理等,针对不同等级的护理服务给予不同的支付比例,引导有序的护理服务。目前,上海市长期护理保险适用于职工医保和 60 周岁及以上城乡居民医保参保人员,试点期内由单位按缴费基数的 1% 缴纳职工长期护理保险费,居保人员由个人承担 15% 左右的参保费用。随着长期护理保险的逐步推进,有必要在考虑本市经济社会发展和基金实际运行情况的基础上,综合考虑人口结构、医疗费用、护理费用、行业发展等因素的共同影响,建立多方动态筹资机制。

(二)构建激励约束机制,确保筹资效率

卫生筹资政策应保证一系列系统性的激励来促进综合性卫生服务,而不鼓励对孤立的单独事件做出临时反应①。具体来看,可通过优化供需双方的共同资源配置,提高资金使用效率。

针对需方,可通过发挥保险的杠杆作用,在广泛开展技术评估、政策干预经济学分析的基础上,针对老年人的常见病、多发病等,拉大不同等级医院的支付比例差距,引导老年人有序就医。对开展综合性评估、实施能延缓或防止功能衰退的预防措施以及支持长期照护(包括康复、姑息治疗和临终关怀)的医疗机构给予经济激励。

针对供方,除加大为老年人提供医疗服务的医务人员报酬支付力度外,还应该保证为老年人提供预防、慢病管理、康复服务的社区和初级卫生保健机构的工作人员也能获得相应激励。此外,应结合支付制度改革等措施,理顺卫生服务体系,如在上海已经推行的"1+1+1"医联体签约试点政策内医疗机构实行总额预算和打包付费,试点家庭医生实行按人头支付方式,通过确定各级医疗机构适宜提供的医疗服务清单,设定不同级别医疗机构的支付标准,强化各级医疗机构开展本级机构所应提供的服务的能力,并制定宣传策略②,做好政策解读。

---

① 世界卫生组织.关于老龄化与健康的全球报告,2016.http://www.who.int/ageing/publications/world-report-2015/zh/.

② 世界银行集团、世界卫生组织、财政部、国家卫生和计划生育委员会、人力资源社会保障部.健康中国深化中国医药卫生体制改革建设基于价值的优质服务提供体系政策总论,2016.

二、转型服务提供模式，发展适老的整合型服务

随着上海市居民健康水平的提升，人均期望寿命不断增长，疾病谱和死因谱逐渐发生改变，"以疾病为中心"的传统医学模式正在被"以人为中心"的"生物—心理—社会"医学模式所取代，老年人群对医疗卫生服务的需求也日益多样化。这就要求政策制定者根据老年人的特点，发展以老年人为中心的、整合型的服务模式。

（一）以老年人为中心提供服务

上海市老年人慢性疾病、共患疾病发生率高，2015年上海市老年人中，因4种及以上疾病就诊的人数约占总就诊人数的一半。慢性疾病需要长期、定期接受治疗，同时共患病要求多管齐下，还要开展康复服务，防止或延缓因疾病导致的失能失智。目前上海市老年人的医疗服务模式仍以急性期疾病治疗为主，就诊行为常发生在多个医疗机构，存在着严重的医疗记录不连贯和医疗服务碎片化现象。根据英国经验，需从以下几个方面分阶段逐步建立以老年人为中心的服务模式。

一是医疗资源逐步向社区及健康促进转移。 控制公立医院规模，不再扩张床位，把更多的人力、物力投入社区卫生服务，注重居民行为和生活方式的干预，提高其对健康的正确认识，减轻或消除影响健康的危险因素。

二是基于需要提供服务。 向英国整合型服务路径（Integrated Care Pathway）学习，筛选出老年人的重点疾病与重点人群（如高龄老人），通过对其身体状况、家庭支持等方面进行综合评估确定优先需要，以此建立一系列标准化的整合型服务路径，包括诊断标准、服务标准、转诊标准、预防服务等。

三是发展个性化服务方案。 推行多学科综合治疗（Multi-disciplinary Team，MDT）模式，实现以患者为中心的个性化服务。根据老年人个体制定有针对性的、个性化的服务包，由固定的多学科服务团队提供服务并进行健康管理。

（二）建立整合型的服务模式

整合型的服务模式不仅基于社区，更需要对医疗卫生体系进行统筹考虑、整体整合。整合的形式可分为以下几个层次。

一是水平整合。 此处包括同级医院、养老机构、老年护理机构等涉老服务

机构间的沟通合作,还包括医疗卫生、社会服务等服务间的有机结合。可建立卫生部门与民政、医保、残联等政府部门的联席会议制度,设置整合型服务管理决策层负责协调。

二是纵向整合。完善分级诊疗,落实各级医疗机构功能定位和健康守门人制度,逐步实施社区首诊和双向转诊,包括长处方、健康管理、优先转诊、开放部分三级医院专家号源、上级医院延续用药等一系列优惠政策和服务,保证患者在预防、诊断、治疗、康复、功能恢复与生活能力提高等方面的连续性。探索建立专科联盟,利用三甲医院的技术优势支持基层医疗卫生机构,实现资源共享。目前上海市正在推行的"1+1+1"医联体签约试点即为探索之一。

三是机构内部整合。在基层医疗卫生机构,加快对中医医师、社区护士、康复治疗师、营养师、心理咨询师和社会工作者等专业人员的培养和培训,加强以全科医生为核心的多学科服务团队建设;在综合性医疗卫生机构,由多学科专家共同为老年患者会诊,为老年患者就诊提供综合的诊疗服务。

四是预防和治疗服务整合。服务方式从以疾病治疗为主导转向治疗和预防相结合,同时关注影响老年人群的社会和心理因素,以社区为载体,对老年人开展全面、全程、有针对性的健康管理。此外,因老少分居、空巢家庭带来的老年人的孤独感,以及社会压力导致的精神疾病等问题,对老年人群健康的影响不可忽视。在服务提供过程中需同时强调精神卫生方面的防控。

五是医生和患者整合。英国经验表明,病人参与和自主性(patient involvement and independence)是非常重要的。从供方来看,要配合居民签约、分级诊疗和社区家庭医生制度的实施,鼓励老年人群参与健康管理和医疗决策过程,增进医患信任;从需方来看,要加强健康教育和舆论引导,帮助患者从正规途径获知正确的健康知识,为自身健康承担更多的责任。

六是医疗服务和社会服务的整合。英国经验表明,通过整合原本分割的医疗服务体系与社会服务体系,为居民提供一站式(one-stop)服务,有利于提高资源利用效率和整体服务质量。在以全科医生为中心的社区基层医疗团队基础上,融合社会服务工作人员,双方相互配合,组成区域性健康维护网络。

由英国经验可知,整合型的服务模式对于资源的利用更加有效,能在一定程度上改善老年人健康结果。建立以老年人为中心的、整合型的服务模式,加强以全科医生为核心的多学科服务团队建设,探索基于需要的个性化服务方案,推动卫生服务与社会服务的有机统筹,是应对上海市人口老龄化挑战的有效途径之一。

三、加强资源配置规划,强调统筹、整合和优化

在上海市人口老龄化日益凸显的同时,老年人的照护问题越来越突出,涉老服务资源供给不足已成为制约老年照护发展的关键因素[①],主要体现在三个方面。一是医护人员数量严重短缺[②]。床位、医护人员和照护人员数量缺口大,不能满足需求。二是照护质量参差不齐。部分机构配置不佳,照护人员文化水平偏低、职业服务期短、流失率高。三是资源错配。上海市涉老服务资源和水平在各个区域和机构之间分布、发展不均衡,床位空置和"压床"现象并存,社会居家养老和养老机构缺乏足够的医疗支持[③]。为破除这三大掣肘因素,需从几方面多管齐下、多措并举。

(一) 在布局规划上,落实基于大数据的涉老服务资源配置规划

《上海市养老设施布局专项规划(2013—2020 年)》和《上海市老年医疗护理服务体系规划(2016—2020 年)》明确提出增加老年护理服务资源供给。首先,根据区域内人口社会学特征,医疗机构、养老机构和社区居家服务机构分布,就诊患者来源等信息,建立大数据网络。其次,基于大数据,统筹协调区域内老年医疗、护理和康复等资源配置,将涉老服务整合纳入区域功能规划与建设中。同时,落实科学的资源配置规划,鼓励制定区域规划时整合和扩增资源,充分调动与利用存量和增量资源,调整各级各类机构的结构布局,为老年人提供多样化、全方位、系统性的服务。

(二) 在资金利用上,通过长期护理保险促进资源统筹

上海市作为全国首批 15 个长期护理保险制度试点城市之一,于 2017 年

---

① 张强,高向东.老年人口长期护理需求及影响因素分析——基于上海调查数据的实证分析[J].西北人口,2016(2)：87—90.
② 丁汉升,杜丽侠,赵薇,等.上海市老年护理需求、费用及存在问题研究[J].老龄科学研究,2014(2)：47—53.
③ 焦翔,侯佳乐,田卓平.上海市老年护理供需测算与长期护理制度建设研究[J].中国医院管理,2014,34(7)：24—29.

1月在徐汇、普陀、金山三个区先行开展长期护理保险试点工作①。从供方来看,通过长期护理保险的支持,不论医疗机构、养老机构或社会居家养老服务机构,只要符合资质,其提供的医疗卫生、照护服务和社会服务将一并纳入保险支付范围。长期护理保险打破了医疗、养老分属不同主管部门的樊篱,将资金池进行统筹利用。随着试点的推进,服务清单项目将进一步扩大。从需方来看,长期护理保险增强了老年人养老服务购买能力。一方面能够刺激市场,吸引各类经营主体平等参与、共享经费;另一方面,活力迸发的市场将提供多种多样的服务,充分满足老年人多层次的需求。同时,资金方面不仅需要长期护理保险,更重要的是医疗保障资金的支持和激励。通过医保支付方式改革,完善正向激励的支付体系,鼓励医务人员提供恰当的服务,引导老年人去接受恰当的服务。

(三) 在机构资源上,推动医疗机构、养老机构多种形式的结合与调整

推进医疗机构和养老机构结合,已有如下几种形式。

一是养老机构设置医疗机构。上海市政府分别于 2015 年、2016 年将"新增 50 家养老机构设置医疗机构"纳入市政府实事项目。卫生部门积极指导符合审批条件的养老机构设置医疗机构,并制定下发了《上海市养老机构设置医疗机构工作指南》。

二是医疗机构开设养老机构。卫生部门鼓励医疗机构托管或开设养老机构,支持其享受民政部门对养老机构的床位建设补贴和每月运营补贴等优惠政策。

三是医疗机构和养老机构合作。首先,社区卫生服务中心与养老服务机构合作。上海市制定了《社区卫生服务中心与养老服务机构签约服务规范》,积极推进社区卫生服务中心与养老服务机构建立签约合作服务模式。2015 年底,养老机构与医疗机构签约率达 100%。其次,社区托养机构与医疗机构合作。依托现有的社区老年日间照护中心、社区生活服务中心等社区托养机构,由护理站或社区卫生服务中心会同社工、志愿者上门提供医疗护理等服务。2016 年底,社区托养机构与医疗机构签约率为 64%,2017 年底达到 100%。

---

① 上海市人民政府.市政府关于印发《上海市长期护理保险试点办法》的通知. http://www.shanghai.gov.cn/nw2/nw2314/nw2319/nw12344/u26aw51124.html[2016-12-29].

四是利用社区卫生服务中心平台整合涉老服务资源。 社区卫生服务中心提供的六大类 141 项基本服务项目中，69 项以老年人群为主要服务对象，社区护理、居家护理、老年人健康管理、舒缓疗护服务等占其总工作量的 57%。

同时，鼓励部分一二级医院转型为老年护理院，鼓励综合医院开展老年护理床位转换。对于设置老年护理床位的区县综合性医院，通过福利彩票公益金给予每张床位 1 万元的一次性补助。此外，动员社会力量参与社会养老服务，特别关注重点老年人群如低收入、高龄、独居、失能、失智老年人等，鼓励和支持社会力量兴办涉老服务机构，鼓励志愿者组织、公益慈善组织开展形式多样的老年人关爱服务活动。

（四）在人员队伍上，培育建设从业队伍

目前我国对于护理员还没有形成规范的职业准入、培训和评价体系，导致人才队伍良莠不齐。而老年人群对照护服务需求大、增长快，需要从资源规划出发，加快从业人员队伍建设，可由以下几点入手。

一是开发护理员职业系列。《全国护理事业发展规划（2016—2020）》提出"加快护理员队伍建设"。可探索将养老护理员、医院护工（护理员）、家政服务员等几支队伍进行整合，统一合并为国家或地方"养老护理员"，并设职业资格证书。

二是建立护理员培养途径。 首先，需要出台护理员准入标准、职业标准、教育标准、评价标准等一系列指导文件。其次，完善护理员梯队的培训、认证、上岗体系。可根据其执业地和工作内容的不同，设计不同培训学时与内容。再次，完善护理员继续教育，在职护理员需要定期更新职业资质，鼓励低中级护理员通过培训考试后获取高等级证书。

三是提高护理员待遇。 建设规模适度、结构合理的护理员人才梯队，等级越高的护理员给予越高的收入。

资源合理配置不可能一蹴而就，要从规划、实施、评价等各个环节一一落实完善。上海市在医养结合方面已经先行先试，做出了一系列有意义的探索，需要保持科学规划和顶层设计的优势，强调现有资源的统筹、整合和优化，积极、稳妥地推进各项措施的落实。

四、促进医疗服务合理利用，有效控制医疗费用

我国在经济尚不发达的情况下提前进入老龄社会，属于"未富先老"。医

疗费用随着老年人口数量的增长而急剧增长。同时由于劳动力减少,医保基金的收入平衡也受到严峻考验。老年人群患病多、药费高,费用难以控制,监管也存在一定困难。

(一)重点监测不合理医疗服务利用

在控制浪费方面,监测医疗费用过高、门急诊次数过多、住院次数过多、住院天数过长的人群。研究发现,2015 年,上海市老年人口组与其他年龄组医疗资源消耗倍数关系与国际一般经验相符,但高年龄段人口的服务利用和费用均呈现"翘尾",生命表模型分析结果显示,上海市老年人口医疗费用支出相对较高,提示存在不合理利用。临终前患者中,16%的患者人均医疗费用超过 15万,占样本人群临终前总医疗费用的一半。医疗费用最大值为 405.51 万元,其中 1%的患者(约 500 人)的累计医疗费用达到 4.16 亿(人均 83 万),5%的患者(约 2 500 人)累计医疗费用达到 10.85 亿元(人均 43 万)。住院费用的回归分析结果显示,住院天数是主要的影响因素之一①。针对临终前费用的临近死亡效应,本次调查中,病例持续时间最长的为全年住院,把医院当成了"疗养院"。在单次住院天数超过 180 天的患者中,有 50.11%的住院机构为社区卫生服务中心,21.29%的为护理院,5.63%为精神病医院,仍有超过 16%的患者在综合医院及中医医院中住院超过 180 天。针对以上问题,建议:

一是监测高额医疗费用,评估医疗服务的合理性和价值。可参照国外经验建立独立的医疗费用审查机制。日本、韩国均成立了独立的医疗费用审查机构,审核成员由保险机构代表、医生代表、患者代表等多方代表组成,审查各医疗机构、各年龄阶段、各病种的费用情况②③。中国台湾地区医疗费用审查由健保局承担,除一般费用审查之外,还抽样进行专业审查,如疾病诊断是否正确、检验检查是否必要、治疗和手术与诊断病情是否一致、用药种类和剂量是否符合规定等④。

二是监测长期住院天数、门急诊次数,合理转诊和分流,防范医疗浪费。应当对可能存在医疗浪费的人员进行监测,确有医疗需求的,应转诊到基层或

---

① 吴怀阳,王财元,郭红霞.影响住院费用若干因素分析[J].中国医院统计,2004,11(2):138—139.

② 翟绍果.韩国国民健康保险费用偿付制度概览[J].中国医疗保险,2012(7):70—72.

③ 吕学静.日本医疗点数付费方式及借鉴[J].中国医疗保险,2010(6):58—59.

④ 丁汉升,杜丽侠,李芬,等.台湾健保总额预付制[R],2012.

使用家庭病床;对于一些难以治愈、治疗效果不明显的疾病,尽量避免长期留院①。在住院时间较长的老年护理院中,通过制定合理的出入院标准,提高老年护理资源的使用效率。临终前 2 年,老年人累计门诊次数最高达到 471 次,相当于每月门诊就医约 20 次;77 人每月门诊就医超 200 次。提示存在严重的医疗浪费,需要深入个案调查了解原因。

三是加强对医疗机构服务行为的监管。上海市医保范围内费用的报销比例实际上已达到较高水平。然而,住院费用数据显示,住院自付费用中,约六成是自负费用,近四成是自费费用。自费项目中,对于成本效果好、与社会经济水平发展相适应的服务项目、药物,应考虑纳入报销范围。对于其他自费项目应加强管控,重点管控老年人口、重点疾病类型的自费费用,利用大数据对各医疗机构的总体自费比例、重点疾病的自费项目和比例进行监测、公示。

(二) 转变医疗服务模式,减少医疗费用支出

上海市医疗服务以疾病为中心、以急症处理为主要内容。现代医学认为,疾病早期预防、早期诊断是提升居民健康水平的最佳服务模式。世界卫生组织也认为,21 世纪的医学将从"疾病医学"向"健康医学"发展,从"重治疗"向"重预防"发展②。《"健康中国 2030"规划纲要》指出,建设健康中国的战略核心是以人民健康为中心,"坚持以基层为重点,预防为主","推动人人参与、人人尽力、人人享有","落实预防为主","强化早诊断、早治疗、早康复"。疾病早期预防、早期诊断具有可观的投资效益。哥伦比亚大学的研究证实,如果加强早期诊断,国家用于疾病的医疗费用将大大减少。以心血管病为例,英国、德国、中国等国用于该病的医疗费用都能减少 42%,美国也能减少 36%(约 1 424 亿美元)。以英国为例,大多数针对老年人的综合医疗服务模型致力于通过人群管理工具来整合临床及其他医疗服务。这些基于人群的模型通过可信的标准化方法将人群分入不同的风险组来实现病例早发现。同时,英国建立了不同的风险预测模型,并为国民医疗服务体系(NHS)的机构所使用。除实现病

---

① 罗仁夏.10 万元以上医疗保险住院病例医疗费用肥西[J].中国卫生资源,2005(6):41—42.

② 王鸿春,马仲良,鹿春江.民生策论:关于转变医疗模式政策的研究[J].资治文摘(管理版),2009(1):62—63.

例早发现以外,这些工具还可用于人群间的资源配置及绩效管理和评价。通过更紧密的医患沟通、更好的预防筛查、更有效的高危病人管理以及高额医疗支出项目的精细化管理,建立一套医疗教育、预防和管理体系,配合常规治疗,长期来看有助于提高医疗治疗效率,合理控制医疗费用。

(三)通过综合干预,避免或延缓入院,及早出院

加强机构合作,采取适当机制,鼓励节约型服务利用模式,减少老年人不合理的住院服务,避免或延缓入院,鼓励老年人接受适当时期和适当内容的服务。英国在基于社区的避免入院机制以及早期出院支持方面的经验,可供其他医疗服务体系借鉴[①]。

现有的医疗服务体系并不能很好地服务于老年患者,在目前尚未建立合理有序的就医秩序的情况下,许多导致人们入院的健康问题实际上在社区就能得到很好的解决,从而避免住院。事实上,西方国家越来越多地建立了社区提供针对急性症状的服务模式。以澳大利亚为例,建立了 Hospital in the Home(HIH)和 Hospital in the Nursing Home (HINH)服务体系[②],在患者家中提供医疗和护理服务,从而避免患者入院。研究显示,作为急性住院服务的替代模式,HIH 和 HINH 对于特定的患者和症状是安全的、可接受的、富有效率的。为了实现这种服务模式,机构之间必须建立有效的转诊机制和沟通策略。随着人群老龄化程度的加深,降低老年护理院患者的入院率对于提高患者健康结果有着重要的意义,能够降低医院获得性并发症,并且能让老人在熟悉的环境中接受医疗服务。

(四)发挥护理、康复对急症治疗的替代作用

研究发现,我国老年护理院"压床"现象严重。大量仅需要低密度医疗护理的老年人群选择进入医疗机构养老,甚至有一些老人在医院的老年病区或老年医院享受长期护理服务,利用现有的医疗保险为长期护理付费。也有报道表示,由于医保的作用,老人们认为"地段医院比养老院更实惠",故想"借"

---

① Pramod Prabhakaran,SHDRC Report:UK integrated care perspective (Draft),2017.

② Crilly J,Chaboyer W,Wallis M. A structure and process evaluation of an Australian hospital admission avoidance programme for agedcare facility residents.Journal of Advanced Nursing,2012,68(2):322—334.

医院床位养老①。事实上，没有治疗价值的老年人住院治疗，对医疗保险体系是巨大威胁。医疗保险的参保人员常常以医疗护理的需求把照护服务的成本带入医疗保险和医疗救助。尽管医保基金支付这些费用是合法的，但却很不经济②，这种服务的不合理转移，挤占了有限、昂贵的医疗资源，人为地造成了看病难的现象。国际经验发现，护理及康复对住院服务有很大的补充替代作用，更能对老龄患者的精神心理护理带来远期裨益。建议推动舒缓疗护（临终关怀）项目，设立机构和居家舒缓疗护床位，为老年人在生命末期提供临终关怀。然而，尽管框架体系已经存在，但资源整合尚待发展，护理及康复服务的利用有待提高，亟需相关部门整合医疗服务资源，优化为老养老服务结构。

五、提高公平性，缩小不同制度之间的差异

社会经济环境直接或间接影响着老年人的健康，由于个体特征不同（如家庭出身、性别等），环境对健康的影响存在巨大差异，进而导致卫生不平等和不公平③。尤其是老年人，相当一部分老年人之间存在的能力和现状的巨大差异，很有可能是由其生命过程中所有健康不平等现象所致的累积效应④。实证研究表明，影响医疗服务利用的因素主要有经济水平、健康状况和医疗保障水平等，相关因素的多样性导致医疗服务利用和医疗负担的不公平，进而影响老年人的健康公平⑤⑥。上海市医疗服务利用和费用情况也显示，三大基本医疗保险的筹资标准、报销水平、医疗保障水平差异较大，因此，有必要从筹资和服务利用等多方面入手，促进老年人的健康公平。

①　许燕君,杨颖华,杨光,等.上海市老年护理床位配置现状及问题[J].中国卫生资源,2014(3)：157—159.

②　杨团.中国长期照护的政策选[EB/OL]http：//info.bjxwx.com/a/OlderWorld/OlderIndustry/IndustryNews/2016/1223/34054.html.

③　Commission on Social Determinants of Health.Closing the gap in a generation：health equity through action on social determinants of health. Final report of the Commission on Social Determinants of Health.Geneva：World Health Organization，2008.

④　Dannefer D. Cumulative advantage /disadvantage and the life course：cross-fertilizing age and social science theory [J]. J Gerontol B Psychol Sci Soc Sci，2003，58(6)：S327-37.doi：ttp：//dx.doi.org/10.1093/geronb/58.6.S327 PMID：14614120.

⑤　陈培榕,吴拉,朱丽莎.老年人医疗服务利用及其影响因素分析——基于中国健康与养老追踪调查的数据[J].中国社会医学杂志,2015,32(2)：153—155.

⑥　解垩.与收入相关的健康及医疗服务利用不平等研究[J].经济研究,2009(2)：92—105.

（一）重点保障弱势老年人群健康权益

建议结合重特大疾病保障机制，推进完善老年人健康公平。一是在全面实施城乡居民大病保险基础上，采取降低起付线、提高报销比例、合理确定合规医疗费用报销范围等措施，提高大病保险对困难群众支付的精准性。二是在做好低保对象、特困人员等的医疗救助基础上，将低收入家庭的老年人以及因病致贫家庭的重病患者纳入救助范围，发挥托底保障作用。三是积极引导社会慈善力量等多方参与，形成医疗卫生机构与医保经办机构间的数据共享机制，推动基本医保、大病保险、医疗救助、疾病应急救助、商业健康保险的有效衔接，全面提供一站式服务。

（二）统筹基本医保制度，促进制度公平

2016年起，上海市开始推行城乡居民基本医疗保险管理办法，整合城镇居民医保和新农合，实现了覆盖范围、筹资政策、保障待遇、医保目录、定点管理、基金管理的"六统一"。但对上海市老年人来说，城乡居民基本医保与小城镇医保、职工医保的筹资与保障待遇仍存在差异。建议进一步统筹完善基本医保制度，率先保障各制度间老年人医疗护理服务的公平性，进而保障全人群的公平。具体来看，**一是建立稳定可持续的筹资机制**，在医保缴费参保政策中厘清政府、单位、个人缴费责任，在继续加大财政投入重点向老年人倾斜、提高政府补助标准的同时，强化个人参保意识，适当平衡不同制度间个人缴费比重，如可探索职工医保个人账户结余资助家庭成员（尤其是老年人）参加城乡居民医保。**二是健全与筹资水平相适应的医保待遇动态调整机制**，包括统筹基本医疗保障边界、合理确定基本医保待遇标准等，鼓励基本医保个人账户家庭共济，使家庭中疾病风险和医疗费用相对较低的年轻人能够对老年人进行补贴。**三是提升医保经办管理能力水平**，在药品采购和费用结算、医保支付标准谈判、定点机构的协议管理和结算等方面加大改革创新力度，进一步发挥医保对医疗费用不合理增长的控制作用，促进制度公平。

（三）构建基于结果的健康公平理论框架

全民医疗保险可以改变以往基本医疗保险制度依托的选择性原则和身份歧视等理念，克服客观存在的不同制度人员间的费用转嫁，充分体现普及性、

全民性、平等性、公民权利、基本需要和健康优先等现代福利价值观念①。随着我国全民医保制度的推进，有关健康公平的理论不再是以往有无保障的机会公平，而是基于权利和需求的过程与结果公平，是个人权利底线与政府责任底线的统一。具体来看，公平性分析主要包括水平公平（Horizontal Equity）和垂直公平（Vertical Equity）。以医疗护理保障制度为例，水平公平主要包括三个维度，即广度公平（覆盖率）、宽度公平（保障内容）和高度公平（保障待遇），要求处于相同状况的人得到同样的对待；垂直公平则要求针对不同的医疗服务需求可以提供不同层次的保障包。而这些措施仅能保障过程公平，更重要的是要确保健康结果的公平。构建基于结果的健康公平理论框架，一要明确相关政策执行的目标，从关心投入转向关心产出，进而达到更好的政策结果②，包括提高健康水平、服务品质、病人满意度以及减轻患者经济负担等；二要从老年人需求出发，将医疗费用和护理费用共同纳入补偿范围，根据"同等需要同等对待"原则，通过预防、治疗、康复、护理和临终关怀等体系的衔接整合，促进老年人全程、全面健康公平；三要加大对基本医疗和公共卫生的投入，通过转移支付、倾斜政策等措施优化卫生资源配置，促进过程公平，进而实现老年人健康结果公平。

六、制定靶向减负政策，保护筹资风险

（一）防范重大疾病患者的个人负担风险

按照住院总费用排名，2015 年，上海市老年人组别中，排名前三的疾病类别分别是循环系统疾病、恶性肿瘤、呼吸系统疾病，住院总费用及自付费用均较高。上海市城保建立了综合减负制度、居保设立了大病保险，用以减轻重大疾病患者的医疗负担。纳入大病医保的参保人员的疾病负担得到有效减轻，4 个病种（包括重症尿毒症透析、肾移植抗排异、恶性肿瘤和部分精神病病种）患者的医保补偿比例普遍提高 23～24 个百分点。然而，4 个病种的界定使得纳入保障范围有限，老年人负担重的慢性病如脑卒中等没有纳入，造成重大疾病负担的罕见病也不在大病保险的报销范围内。从资金的充足性和可持续性

---

① 刘继同."一个制度、多种标准"与全民性基本医疗保险制度框架[J].人文杂志，2006(3)：7—13.

② Yip W C，Hsiao W C，Chen W，et al. Early appraisal of China's huge and complex health-care reforms [J].Lancet，2012，379(9818)：833—842.

来看,2015 年,大病医保报销费用占居民医保支出总额的比例为 0.5%;而截至
2016 年,居民医保累计结余 4.1 亿元(占当年基金收入的 17.1%),大病报销占
累计基金结余的 3.2%,仍有大量结余资金沉积。为进一步提高对重大疾病的
保障力度,建议采取以下措施:

**其一,以流行病学、疾病负担数据为基础,逐渐扩大上海市大病保险的病
种范围。**大病保险在 4 类病种基础上,按照病情重、病程长、费用高的原则,逐
步扩大病种范围。针对患大病的困难老年人群,通过制定"靶向"减负政策予
以保障。例如,大病保险范围包括重症尿毒症透析、肾移植抗排异、恶性肿瘤、
部分精神病病种,纳入的病种有限,如老年人口患病率、住院总费用最高的循
环系统疾病没有纳入,建议按照病情重、病程长、费用高的原则,逐步扩大病种
范围。

其二,补充设立按费用界定大病的机制。按照病种界定大病,易操作,
费用较易控制,有利于保障基金运营的安全性;然而许多发生高额医疗费
用的患者不在政策规定的重大疾病之内。按费用界定,即在一定时期内,
当患者发生的医疗费用较高,甚至超出事先规定的高额费用标准时,可将
其所患疾病视为重大疾病。以费用为切入点进行保障,能有效减少参保
人员因病返贫、因病致贫的情况,具有更大的公平性。由于按病种界定的
方式已经对医疗费用负担重的患者有一层保障,按费用界定作为补充方
式,在设立之初,费用标准可适当提高,待筹集资金充足时再调低标准,扩
大保障面。

其三,从长远看,设立自负封顶线。我国的医保支付制度普遍设置医保支
付封顶线而非自负封顶线,这一机制保护的是医保收支平衡,而不是患者疾病
的风险。这一制度造成的后果是低收入人群、罹患重大疾病的人群仍然看不
起病,其应当享受的公共卫生资源被其他人群所利用。建议根据经济发展水
平,划定自负封顶线水平及收入水平线(底线公平),经审查后由统筹基金全额
支付封顶线以上的医疗费用。对于重大疾病、特殊困难人群再予以一定的医
保救助或减免措施。

(二) 通过护理保障与补贴降低非直接医疗费用

通过中国养老与健康追踪抽样数据可以得到我国分年龄段老龄人口中失
能老人的比例,2011 年,60 岁及以上老年人口中失能老人比率约为 16.37%。
随着我国老龄人口的快速增长,有研究预计,到 2030 年,我国失能老人规模将

达到 5 744 万人，由此将产生 2.1 万亿元的庞大老年护理服务需求，占当年 GDP 的 1.7%[1]。然而，由于我国老年人口整体有低收入、低消费的现象，在现阶段可能无法将庞大的老年护理服务需要转换为实际利用需求。历史数据显示，我国老年人口生活来源主要是家庭成员供养、劳动收入以及离退休养老金。即使是保障水平较高的城市老人，其养老金也只能覆盖日常生活支出的76%，难以支付人工成本日趋昂贵的老年护理服务。同时，大部分失能老人的照护服务都无法报销，导致高额的直接非医疗成本。例如，在访谈过程中得知，一位需要长期住院的急性脑梗塞患者，其日夜护工费用达到 210 元/日，这部分费用是需要患者家庭自己承担的，并且这部分隐形成本并没有反映在医疗费用账单里，长期来看将给患者家庭带来沉重的经济负担。目前我国老年人主要以家庭照护为主。然而，部分老人因高龄、慢性病等原因长期处于卧床、半卧床状态，丧失了基本的生活自理能力，从起居活动到吃饭洗浴，完全依赖照料者，这为家庭照料带来了严重的负担；部分照料者（Care Giver）自身身体健康状况较差，有的还同时担负着工作和抚养下一代的任务，也使老年人的居家照护面临着十分严峻的挑战。

建议尽快建立提供护理服务费用补偿的长期照护保险制度。同时，在社区和家庭层面，建立完善的社区卫生服务体系，建立起医院—社区—家庭的综合关怀支持系统，确保失能老年人和照顾者能得到充分的社区医疗、健康服务资源，教育家庭其他成员从不同层面分担照顾者工作，给予照顾者精神上的支持和物质或体力上的帮助，帮助照顾者重视自身健康与照顾工作的关系，给予照顾者更多情感和精神上的支持[2]。此外，通过财政或保险为家庭照护人员提供护理补贴，促进家庭养老，减轻家庭照护者的经济负担。

七、发展社会服务，注重人文关怀

英国的医疗卫生服务与社会服务分属卫生部和地区政府（Local Authority）两个不同的政府部门管理，历史上存在服务不连贯的问题。我国和上海市也面临着同一挑战，医疗卫生和养老服务分属卫生和民政两个部门，

---

① 袁文蔚.我国老年护理消费需求与购买力分析[D].北京：清华大学,2013.
② 何香,朱海萍,刘华玲,等.失能老年人照顾者护理负担的研究[J].中国护理管理,2014(5)：503—505.

服务提供和支付在衔接上有一定难度,为老年人群带来了诸多不便。2013 年
10 月,《国务院关于加快发展养老服务业的若干意见》(国发〔2013〕35 号)中第
一次明确提出医养结合发展的概念,上海市人民政府于 2014 年 4 月发布的
《关于加快发展养老服务业推进社会养老服务体系建设的实施意见》(沪府发
〔2014〕28 号)中也指出"推进社会养老服务体系建设",以期能满足老年人多样
化的需求。

(一) 统筹社会服务,推动社会养老服务体系发展

2002 年,英国 NHS 引入整合保健信托(Integrated Care Trusts)来提供更
好的、整合的医疗卫生与社会服务。目前一些地区正在试点将卫生服务和社
会服务的预算进行合并,并对管理架构进行整合,在社区层面实现卫生和社会
服务的统一管理①。建议可按照以下几方面来发展社会服务。

生活方面,为老年人群提供的社会服务,不仅要以满足其生活需求为目
的,还要通过为其服务降低危险因素、减轻疾病负担、减少急诊和住院,进而节
约资源,提高健康水平;此外,针对部分老年人群重点需要的服务,积极争取财
政部门支持,以市政府实事项目等形式进行推进。例如,可借鉴日本已纳入长
期护理保险的辅助用具租赁、住宅无障碍化改造等社会服务项目,学习借鉴目
前各大城市非常流行的公共自行车租赁运行方式,试点失能老人辅助用具租
赁,进行分区域、分步骤地推广。

社区方面,通过上海市 16 个区正在推进的老年照护统一需求评估,统筹
协调区域内服务资源。可在社区层面联合委任一位或多位整合型服务体系管
理者,负责整个社区医疗卫生与社会服务的管理沟通。

社会方面,发展社会服务不仅需要政府主导,还要呼吁家庭、社会的共同
参与。治理理论倡导政府与社会组织以及其他社会力量的协作互动、合作共
治,以实现公共利益的最大化②。通过鼓励社会组织提供社会服务,能够有效
统筹整合社会上分散的服务资源,提高服务效率。

发展方向上,英国部分地区已经实现了卫生服务和社会服务的预算整合,

---

① Ham C,de Silva D.Integrating care and transforming community services:What
works? Where next? (Policy Paper)〔R〕.Birmingham:Health Service Management
Centre,University of Birmingham,2009.

② 周耀虹.社区社会组织参与社会服务的途径与价值探析〔R〕.社会管理法治化理论
与实践研讨会,2012.

而目前在上海市，各政府部门之间的樊篱较难打破。可以借由正在试点的长期护理保险计划，制定老年人群最核心需求的社会养老服务项目清单，从支付层面上对社会服务进行支持。发展社会服务不能仅从民政主管部门入手，参考英国经验，需要加强卫生、民政、医保等部门的联动，将社会服务发展融入整体的社会养老服务体系发展中去。

（二）加强社会支持，探讨适宜的临终关怀模式

2004 年，英国推出"临终关怀计划"，并于 2008 年制定全英国范围内的实施策略（End of Life Care Strategy）[1]。政府注重从顶层设计上搭建临终关怀体系，多次对临终关怀领域开展深入调查，同时提出 2015—2020 年舒缓疗护 / 临终关怀总体目标[2]。上海市开展临终关怀工作的主要途径之一是开设舒缓疗护（临终关怀）床位，2012 年、2014 年以市政府实事项目的形式深入推进，目前上海市共有 76 家医疗机构（以社区卫生服务中心为主），共开设居家和机构舒缓疗护床位 1 700 余张，为有需求的老年人和临终患者提供姑息治疗和护理服务。根据英国经验，临终关怀体系在尊重生命的同时，有助于节省医疗成本，提升卫生绩效。构建更适宜的临终关怀模式有以下两点。**一是探索建立家庭—社区—医护人员相结合的临终关怀模式**[3]。识别判断出具备临终关怀需求的末期老人和终末期患者，充分尊重其本人和家属的知情权与选择权。对于选择在基层舒缓疗护床位度过生命最后阶段的老人和患者，形成家庭、社区、医护人员相互协调，各司其职的机制。**二是生理关怀与心理关怀并重。**一方面，临终关怀运用医疗技术缓解躯体痛苦，帮助患者平静离世；另一方面，注重心灵关怀和精神引导。对于有信仰的人，可通过宗教使之正确面对死亡。临终关怀不仅针对老年人和终末期患者，还包括家属。需要教育家属树立正确的生死观，帮助其在合理治疗与传统孝道之间做出权衡，合理使用医疗资源，提高生命末期质量。

老年人群的疾病治疗、缓解痛苦和心理疏导、人文关怀同样重要，社会服

---

[1]　Department of Health.End of Life Care Strategy：Promoting high quality care for adults at the end of their life[R].2008.

[2]　National Palliative and End of Life Care Partnership.Ambitions for palliative and end of life care：A national framework for local action 2015—2020[EB/OL].http：//endoflifecareambitions.org.uk/[2016-12-8].

[3]　陈春燕，罗羽，谢容.当前我国临终关怀模式存在的问题及对策[J].护理管理杂志，2005,5(2)：26—28.

务应与医疗卫生服务有机结合，共同保障老年人安享晚年。临终关怀是整个医疗卫生体系中不可或缺的一环，可从全市层面构建临终关怀体系，明确总体目标，为完善医疗卫生服务体系、节约医疗资源、提高体系运行效率奠定基础。

八、借助信息化大数据，开发基于老年人的健康管理工具

针对老年医疗护理行业面临的海量数据和非结构化数据的挑战，大数据分析有助于提高医疗效率，创造附加价值，获得事半功倍的效果。2015年，国务院发布《促进大数据发展行动纲要》，提出推进医疗大数据的开放共享和汇聚整合，正是希望改变当前老年医疗护理行业存在的数据孤岛、服务割裂现象，通过消除信息技术障碍和数据共享障碍，整合以机构为中心的系统架构，开发以老年人为中心的多元化数据管理工具，应用数据分析结果，积极应对老龄化。

（一）完善数据采集，加强不同组织间数据共享

上海市卫生大数据平台建设主要依托上海市卫生计生委信息中心，启动了以市民健康管理为核心的健康信息网工程，基本形成了"1＋18"个互联互通的数据中心（市中心＋医联＋17个区中心）。实现老年人医疗护理信息的交换和共享，首先要打破跨系统的交互性限制，打通不同组织间的数据壁垒，主要包括：打破公安、卫生、社会保障、民政、残联等多部门"碎片化"数据采集现状，纵向连接市、区两级平台，实现数据的定时传送。在此之前，数据集成部门应制定统一的信息采集标准或规范，使用统一数据传输工具，以确保从不同渠道收集的老年人信息能被唯一识别和二次利用，花大力气提高数据质量。如英国的国家病历中心（Spine）是NHS病人资料的数据库，储存着病人的姓名、性别、年龄、家庭住址等基本信息及病历档案等。延展的国家病历中心还储存了病人的用药、过敏史、药物不良反应等信息，这些信息在紧急时刻可通过网络迅速传递到需要的地点，医护人员可在授权的情况下查看病人档案。通过诸如电子处方服务（Electronic Prescription Service）、汇总护理记录（Summary Care Records）、电子转诊服务（e-Referral Service）等，国家病历中心使信息得以安全地共享①。此外，值得注意的是，当前信息采集仅纳入了公

---

① 　NHS Digital.Spine.https：//digital.nhs.uk/spine.

立医疗机构，尚未连接私营机构如养老院等，更未将主要由家人提供的非正式照护考虑在内。在提倡居家养老护理的背景下，揽入这部分数据可能是今后改革需要考虑的地方。

（二）开发多样化的风险分层工具，推进老年护理评估

当前，大多医疗卫生机构倾向于投入资金用于提高内部的管理效率，很少将患者纳入自身信息化领域范围，尚未将大数据分析结果运用于老年人的医疗护理服务。依托先进的信息技术和海量大数据，开发基于人群的管理工具，可有效利用已有信息，使老年医疗护理更加高效、更加精准、更加个性化。在致力于为老年人群提供整合型、"一体化"医疗护理服务的背景下，利用医院和社区卫生保健数据，开发一套可靠、标准的风险分层工具（Risk Stratification Tools）。根据实时变动的风险分值（Risk Score），医护人员可判断特定一段时间内的高危人群，预测哪些老年人群的风险指数在增加。除标记高风险群体，使之得到尽早管理以外，这些管理工具还能有效支持医疗护理资源在不同老年群体中的合理分配，促进绩效管理和评价。如英国设立了专门针对老年痴呆的数据提取（Dementia Data Extract）项目，旨在从全科医生的日常实践中搜集老年人信息，以此找出可能患有老年痴呆的风险人群。同时，该项目也提取了已确诊老年痴呆患者的就诊信息和其所接受到的服务等。通过统一的评估工具，全科医生对老年人实施专业评估并保持及时跟踪，以确保疾病的早期发现和干预[①]。上海市应用数据管理工具的案例之一是目前正在推进的老年照护统一需求评估。该评估面向老年人群开展，收集的主要信息包括调查对象及其家庭情况、基本生活能力、智力状态、情绪状况、精神状况和疾病诊断等，以期按照评估结果将老年人进行分级，根据其实际需要，适度地、有针对性地提供不同级别的老年照护服务。

（三）依托信息技术，加快推进大数据分析和应用

健康是一个综合、连续的概念，老年阶段作为人生命里程的后期，其健康状况与各阶段的病史都有密切关系。因此，对老年人提供的医疗护理服务也应是可追溯的。推进大数据分析，可在前期加强数据共享和管理的基础上，建

---

① NHS Digital. Dementia data extract. https：//digital. nhs. uk /GP-Collections / service-information/dementia-data-extract.

立相对全面、持续更新的电子健康档案,帮助医护人员掌握老年人各阶段的健康信息。对电子健康档案进行深入分析,有助于进一步确定哪些老年人群是某类疾病的易感人群,帮助医护人员更好地实施照护监控并提供有预测性的服务。同时,电子健康档案也可帮助老年人在既有的健康管理方案中找到最适当的照护方案。电子健康档案应是可移动、可编辑的,便于患者本身及照护者获得。此外,得益于信息技术的发展,加速推进大数据应用,利用远程医疗监护和在线医疗服务,老年慢性病患者可使用高科技智能服装和可穿戴设备,获得远程疾病监护服务。老年人可和全科医生进行在线视频咨询、获取处方,查看完整电子健康档案,借此解放医疗资源,实现老年人健康状态的自我监护,在一定程度上节省健康资源的投入。

总之,有效应对老龄化应充分挖掘大数据背后的潜在价值,对数据进行标准化整合,使之可以共享和比较。依托数据、信息和技术手段,强调基于人群的现代管理方式,研发有价值的风险分层工具,科学评估老年人的健康状况,根据评估结果实行人群分流,有差别地为老年人提供不同类型和深度的医疗护理服务,助力老年人医疗护理资源的合理配置及保障待遇的政策设计,促进慢病和养老服务的健康可持续发展。

九、开展专项战略,应对重点疾病和伤害

针对老年人发病率高、对身心健康影响大的疾病,建立专项战略。

(一) 老年痴呆症战略

根据 2015 年世界阿尔茨海默病报告[①],全球有 4 600 万人患有老年痴呆,该人数大于西班牙整个国家的人口,而到了 2050 年,老年痴呆症患者人数将超过 1.3 亿。在我国,2010 年,65～69 岁老年人患有老年痴呆的比例为2.6%,95～99 岁的老年人中,该病比例将达到 60.5%[②]。分析表明,以往

---

① Alzheimer's Disease International, World Alzheimer Report 2015—The global impact of dementia: An analysis of prevalence, incidence, cost and trends [EB/OL]. https://www.alz.co.uk/research/WorldAlzheimerReport2015.pdf.

② Chan K Y, Wang W, Wu J J, et al.Epidemiology of Alzheimer's disease and other forms of dementiain China, 1990—2010: A systematic review and analysis [J]. Lancet, 2013,381(9882): 2016—2023.

基于小样本的疾病负担研究可能低估了我国老年痴呆症的疾病负担，老年痴呆症的疾病负担增长速度比国际社会预计得更快，政府需要采取迅速有效的应对措施来解决中低收入国家的老年痴呆症问题。首先，应当提高公众对于老年痴呆症的认识，建立有尊严、自主和包容的社会支持系统。第二，提高服务可及性，建立"任务共享"的服务模式，将大部分护理服务下沉到基层护理以及社区服务过程中，由非专业人士经过专业人士培训并在其支持下开展服务。第三，控制危险因素。针对老年痴呆症的危险因素进行分析，最有可能的危险因素是早期的中低教育水平、中年患有高血压以及整个生命过程中的吸烟行为和糖尿病史[1]。越来越多的研究表明，老年痴呆症的风险是可以降低的，同时需要开展更多研究以及健康促进行动[2][3]。开展老年痴呆症危险因素控制的第一步，是让更多人知道，老年痴呆症在某种程度上是可以预防的。最后，应当重视患者家庭服务，因为这可能对人们的健康产生积极影响，并减少给社会带来的成本。同时，发展医疗辅助技术以及上门服务，延缓患者入院。

（二）预防跌倒专项战略

跌倒是 75 岁左右人群致残的主要原因、致死的首要因素，也是许多国家服务框架中规定的对老年人必须关注的首要问题[4]。每年约有 42 万人死于跌倒，其中超过 80% 发生在中低收入国家。预防跌倒以及支持老年人重新获得独立生活的能力，对很多卫生和社会服务组织来说一直是项挑战。预防跌倒专项战略应强调健康教育和培训，创造更安全的环境，优先考虑与跌倒有关的研究，并制定有效政策以减少风险。

---

① Prince M，Albanese E，Guerchet M，et al. World Alzheimer report 2014. Dementia and risk reduction.An analysis of protective and modifiable risk factors.London：Alzheimer's Disease International，2014.

② Lincoln P，Fenton K，Alessi C，et al.The Blackfriars consensus on brain health and dementia [J].Lancet，2014，383(9931)：1805—1806.

③ Norton S，Matthews F E，Barnes D E，et al. Potentialfor primary prevention of Alzheimer's disease：An analysis of population-based data [J]. Lancet，2014，13(8)：788—794.

④ Department of Health.National service framework for older people[EB/OL]. [2015-12-21].http：//www.gov.uk/government/uploads/system/uploads/attachment_data/file/198033/National_Service_Framework_for_Older_People.pdf.

专栏 1　英国的预防跌倒服务自 2004 年开始实施,牛津郡将 Radcliffe 医院所提供的急诊服务与社区卫生和志愿者组织提供的服务整合起来,降低了该郡老年人跌倒的发生率,提高了发生跌倒的老年人以及高风险人群的生命质量。这种模式将多个不同学科领域的专业技能整合到了一起,形成了一个多学科的服务团队,包括:急诊服务、物理治疗师、职业治疗师、跌倒相关专业护士、运动协调专业人士。所提供的服务包括:对养老院员工的培训;对跌倒损伤开展评估;在所有的卫生和社会服务相关领域提高人们对于跌倒的了解和关注;张贴提供跌倒损伤诊疗的机构和服务团队的信息;在社区和医院为老年人提供相关咨询和锻炼项目;在日间服务机构提供有关身体平衡和安全的项目;为高风险人群提供预防性措施的项目;在急诊医院专业团队的支持下,为相关服务人员提供不间断的技术支持和建议;与急救服务合作,通过提供转诊、跌倒预防以及降低拨打急救服务电话频率等方式提高对于跌倒者的保健服务质量。这种服务的转诊可以来源于多个方面,包括服务利用者及其亲属或照顾者。对于个体的特殊需要给予以人为中心、量体裁衣式的服务回应,可以根据具体情况将老年人转诊到体育锻炼项目、职业治疗协助、心理治疗、平衡和安全小组、日间医院治疗或转回全科医生等服务项目中去。

(三)帕金森病战略

我国正处于帕金森病患病人数急剧上升阶段,排除帕金森病患病率的变化,人口老龄化是最重要的原因。2007 年的一项研究结果显示,在目前和今后一段时间内,中国帕金森病患病人数将占全球半数左右。2005 年,中国帕金森病病例数约为 1.99×10^6 例,全球约 4.10×10^6 例;预计到 2030 年,中国帕金森病病例数约 4.94×10^6 例,全球约 8.67×10^6 例[①]。首先,应当建立以证据为基础的帕金森病治疗指南,通过开发和推广指南、评估卫生技术并进行决策转化、开展相关培训和推广等工作,帮助专业人士采用

---

① 刘疏影,陈彪.帕金森病流行现状[J].中国现代神经疾病杂志,2016(2):98—101.

更规范更适宜的卫生技术，从而为居民提供更好的医疗卫生服务。其次，筛选专业人员，构建专业服务局域网，筛选纳入专业水平高且积极性高的医疗及医保专业人员，患者可以向其咨询长期治疗建议。纳入人员包括神经病学家、家庭护理专家、康复专家、精神病专家、心理学家、药剂师、专业的帕金森病护士、行为治疗家、谈话/语言治疗师、营养师及社工等。再次，引入互联网技术，建立健康服务平台。利用互联网技术打破当前医疗瓶颈，建立基于全流程管理的慢性病管理知识平台，通过平台帮助慢性病患者及高危人群实现自我管理，提高其慢性病知晓率和控制率，实现精准健康促进。

　　专栏 2　辅助慢性病管理人员管理慢性病患者，促进慢性病防控工作的有效开展，已经成为医疗行业发展的一个趋势。英国 Parkinson's Excellence Network 以大型公立医院的医疗服务为核心，以基层医疗、社区公共卫生服务为基础，整合各级医疗资源打造"线上服务平台"，使各级医疗资源互通联动，切实有效地为帕金森病患者提供优质的卫生服务。荷兰 Parkinson Net 则建立了专门的信息技术平台，包括具有搜索引擎的专门网址，以及针对患者和专业人士的网络论坛，供彼此在该平台上交流。Parkinson Net 提供了一个面向患者的决策支持工具，患者可以通过此链接找到重要的背景信息，例如帕金森病中不同治疗策略的效果及证据，从而使患者参与决策制定。患者还可以在自己家中通过授权的视频链接进行咨询。Parkinson Net 的关键目标之一是改善患者所接受的治疗的质量透明度，因此需要对治疗质量进行公开。例如，Parkinson Atlas（www.Parkinson Atlas.nl）从不同地区 Parkinson Net 的角度展示相关信息，如医疗花费、入住医院或康复中心的入院率、学科间合作的质量。患者论坛则有助于后续治疗质量的提高。例如，患者用"wiki"（一个应用网站，可以让用户与其他人合作来增加、编辑或删除内容）来创建帕金森病带病生存中有用信息的词条，讨论患者对治疗质量的评价，并提供辅助治疗的经验。针对医疗专业人士，Parkinson Net 提供了一个在线论坛，方便网络内的专家互相沟通，便于他们交流经验和新的治疗技术方面的信息。

(四) 脑卒中战略

脑卒中是在老年人群中多发的急性脑血管疾病,因发病率高、死亡率高、致残率高,已引起了医疗卫生界乃至全社会的重点关注。建议进一步结合脑卒中的临床特点,联合多学科、多部门,建立脑卒中防治网络。应充分结合老年人群的特点,有针对性地建立老年人群的脑卒中救治绿色通道。首先,应联合民政部门,大力加强老年人群脑卒中防治知识宣传,倡导健康生活方式,控制脑卒中危险因素,加强对脑卒中预兆症状的识别。对于高血压、糖尿病老年患者等高危人群,应建立专项课题,开展对脑卒中知识的宣传,促进健康管理意识的提升。其次,在院内,应探索建立急性心脑血管疾病患者绿色通道,加强急诊与临床科室间的衔接。当前,因为医疗救治体制的限制,在脑卒中诊疗过程中,科室协同不足,救治及时性有待加强。建议打破以单一学科为主的卒中救治模式,为老年患者提供个体化、规范化的综合诊疗和干预服务。同时,建立由社区到医院再到社区的卒中救治闭环,为高危人群筛查及卒中患者的临床、康复、照护、心理等需求提供整合型服务。此外,针对老年人群的特点,规划设计卒中患者的运送交通通道,进一步提高救治的及时性和康复的便利性。

十、加强配套措施,形成强有力的政府支持

老龄化在我国及各个省市都将不断加剧,成为一种新的社会常态。老年人的健康状况、机能水平不仅仅取决于医疗服务体系,自然环境和社会环境对于健康老龄化也有着重要影响。营造健康老龄化的环境,涉及多个领域和多个社会角色,各级政府和各个部门需要共同行动。"健康中国2030"提出"健康入万策"理念以及养成健康行为、优化健康服务、完善健康保障、发展健康产业、建设健康环境等五大重点任务,正是引导各个部门、各个领域加强协作,合力促进全民健康水平的提升。

(一) 从四个层面加强各个领域的协同作用

上海市成立了社会养老服务体系建设领导小组办公室,对老龄事业的发展进行统筹协调,指导部门间、区域间的合作,协同应对老龄化,包括建立目标任务、明确责任划分、保障预算以及制定部门间的协作、监测、评估和报告机

制。合作的开展可分为几个层面。**首先,政府部门间的横向合作,**即同级政府不同部门(机构)之间跨越职责和权限合作。如进行老年医疗机构、养老机构的规划、建设,需要规土部门与卫生行政部门进行协作;投放适老小型设施(如易于老年人使用的洗手间、步行通道)需要民政与路政、质监、老龄委协调。**其次,政府部门间的纵向合作,**即市、区两级政府部门就共同的目标、任务开展合作,如落实市级层面统一规划,确保规划落到实处。**第三,政府部门与私营部门的合作,**包括与非政府组织、私营企业、学术机构等的合作。如政府部门与学术机构联合启动老年人健康干预项目,公立医疗机构与私营机构合作开展老年人医疗、照护活动等。**第四,政府与家庭的合作。**例如,政府免费为家庭非正式照护人员提供培训,促进老年人身体机能、生活质量的提高。

(二)建立健康需求导向的资源投入与激励机制

建立结果导向的健康投入机制,开展健康投入绩效监测和评价。世卫报告按照身体机能状况把老年人分为三个阶段:能力强而稳定、能力衰退、能力严重损失。资源、资金投入应注意以下几方面。**首先,保障公共卫生服务,**使老年人不生病、少生病,尽早发现和治疗非传染性疾病。**其次,加大基层卫生投入。**对于患有心血管疾病、肿瘤、慢性呼吸系统疾病、糖尿病和其他非传染性疾病的患者或高危人群,提供有效的疾病管理和卫生服务,防止功能缺陷的累积,降低住院需求,减少使用昂贵的高科技医疗服务。**再次,形成共同目标,加大资金的整合和使用效力。**以养老和医疗的两大主管部门来说,民政部门的救助对象以收入水平为依据,医疗服务需求不是主要关注点;卫生部门则以疾病为出发点,侧重医疗需求,而没有把失能失智老年人的真实需求列为首要工作重点。两个部门安排财政资金时,往往从各自既定的工作重点出发,忽视了以真实需求为导向、更加具有干预成本效果的适宜技术和方法,建议应明确近期和远期的政策目标,采用统一的评估工具开展医疗、护理、照护需求评估,对老年人进行分层服务、精准管理。**最后,应通过优化制度安排实现有限医保资金的精准保障,**最大限度地降低低收入水平、高医疗需求的脆弱老年人的疾病经济负担,通过完善大病医保制度、探索自负封顶线制度,保障合理的医疗护理服务需求。

(三)加强人员培养和培训,加强编制、职业发展支持

老年人疾病的一个重要特点是共患疾病发生率高,上海市 60 岁及以上人口

中,就诊原因为 4 种及以上疾病的人数占到 51.3%,这就决定了老年人多专科联合诊疗的医疗需求。而老年人的健康状况个体差异性大,这一特点决定了其既有疑难杂症诊疗需求,又有长期护理、康复等基本服务需求,医务人员队伍也相应要求既有"顶天"又有"立地"人才,需要研究制定适老医疗服务人员的编制、职业发展、薪酬待遇倾斜性政策,吸引、留住适宜人才。**首先,引进和培养"顶天"人才**。上海市正在建立老年医学中心,要加大针对疑难重症的高层次人才的培养和引进,促进老年医学临床重点学科建设,逐步达到国内乃至国际领先水平。**其次,为老服务关键是要"落地"**。老年人的医疗服务偏重于多专科联合或全科医疗,医务人员的教育及培训要从以急性期疾病治疗为主,转变为慢病管理、以老年人为中心的整体服务视角;特别要加强全科医生培养,提高为老年人提供综合性服务的能力;加强护理、康复等紧缺人员的培养。

（四）通过信息化建设,促进机构间衔接和政府监管

建设好机构数据库,包括为老服务机构的基本信息、医疗服务结构、医疗服务费用等多方面指标,并向社会进行公示。可以参考停车库资源及其利用情况的展示,利用 GIS 技术展示老年人医疗护理资源的分布与服务利用紧张度,有利于患者理性、便捷地选择医疗护理服务机构。建设好个人健康数据库,建立部门间协同的覆盖全人口、全生命周期的健康信息平台,包括个人健康信息、医疗护理需求评估结果、诊疗及处方信息等,实现信息的互联共通,实现公共卫生、医疗服务、医疗保障综合管理等应用信息系统数据集成共享,促进医疗机构间服务有序衔接,使患者得到连续诊疗,提高整体服务效率和效果。对于政府部门,利用"信息＋科技"手段,对服务机构、医务人员服务行为和患者就医行为实行实时、动态监管,监测长期住院天数、高频次门急诊服务和高额医疗费用,评估医疗服务的合理性和价值。

总之,老年阶段是人生命历程中正常且重要的部分。在新的社会经济环境下,老年人口如果能保持较好的健康水平,那么"70 岁即是新的 60 岁",老年人口的角色就可以从被抚养、被照顾者转变为社会效益的创造者,其知识和经验将以多种形式对社会产生益处。面对老龄化这个问题,倡导积极老龄化、健康老龄化,统筹社会、行业和个人三个层面,通过体系优化,借助信息化技术,通过实施应对老龄化的十大策略,预防和减少伤害发生,有效管控慢性病,加大对失能人员的照护,形成维护和促进健康老龄化的强大合力,增加老年人的健康福祉。

第一，拓展筹资渠道，优化筹资机制。加大医保筹资来源，发展长期护理保险，通过设置支付杠杆、改革支付方式，建立激励约束机制。

第二，转型医疗服务模式，以老年人健康为导向，注重对居民行为和生活方式的干预，从横向、纵向、机构内部多个维度建立综合性的医疗服务模式，基于需求，发展个性化的医疗服务。

第三，加强资源配置规划，强调统筹、整合和优化。在布局规划上，落实基于大数据的涉老服务资源配置；在资金利用上，通过长期护理保险促进资源统筹；在机构资源上，推动医疗机构、养老机构多种形式的结合与调整；在人员队伍上，加强人力资源建设，培育从业队伍。

第四，促进医疗服务合理利用，有效控制医疗费用。重点监测不合理医疗服务利用，监测高额医疗费用，监测长期住院天数及门急诊次数，实现合理转诊和分流；通过转变医疗服务模式，减少医疗费用支出；通过综合干预，避免或延缓入院，及早出院；发挥护理、康复对急症治疗的替代作用。

第五，提高公平性，缩小不同制度之间的差异。重点保障弱势老年人群健康权益，统筹基本医保制度，促进制度公平，构建基于结果的健康公平理论框架。

第六，制定靶向减负政策，保护筹资风险。通过扩大大病保险病种、设立自负封顶线，防范重大疾病患者的个人负担过重，通过护理保障与发放财政补贴降低非直接医疗费用。

第七，发展社会服务，注重人文关怀。统筹社会服务，推动社会养老服务体系发展；加强社会支持，探讨适宜的老年临终关怀模式。

第八，借助信息化大数据，开发基于老年人的管理工具。加强不同组织间的数据共享，完善数据采集；依托信息技术，加快推进大数据分析和应用；开发多样化的风险分层工具，推进老年护理评估。

第九，开展专项战略，应对重点疾病和伤害。针对老年人发病率高、对身心健康影响大的疾病，设置老年痴呆症战略、帕金森病战略、脑卒中战略、预防跌倒专项战略等。

第十，加强配套措施，形成强有力的政府支持。统筹老龄事业发展，指导部门间合作，协同应对老龄化，包括建立目标任务，明确责任划分，保障预算，制定部门间的协作，制定监测、评估和报告制度，建立以健康为导向的资源投入与激励机制。

Aging and Medical Expenses: from Mystery to Evidence

CHAPTER ONE   The Framework of Medical Service and Financing System for the Elderly in Shanghai

The demand of medical care of the elderly population is higher than the general population, especially for chronic disease, which has a longer disease course and requires more rehabilitation, nursing and palliative care services. Shanghai's population aging is of high degree and fast speed, which poses a severe challenge to the reactivity of policy-making. Shanghai Municipal Government is very concerned about the issue of aging, focusing on planning for the elderly service system and proceeding to develop the elderly care planning and the security system. This study comprehensively reviewed the policies regarding the provision of medical services and health security for the elderly population in Shanghai, summarized the characteristics and problems of the current system, and proposed suggestions for the future development.

1. Current status of Shanghai health service system for the elderly

The medical service providers in Shanghai are divided into four categories: hospitals, primary health care institutions, public health institutions and other institutions, including both public and non-public institutions. Faced with different kinds of demand of the elderly, i.e., prevention, medical treatment, nursing care and rehabilitation, different kinds of institutions provide relatively targeted health services. Basic treatment, nursing care and rehabilitation for the elderly population are mainly provided by primary health care institutions and medical institutions within nursing homes, including long-term prescriptions for chronic diseases, routine medical examinations and home care. Primary health care institutions also provide training and guidance to the family beds set up at home or nursing homes. In terms of the hospital care and specialized rehabilitation needs of the elderly, it is mainly provided by nursing homes, rehabilitation institutions and medical institutions which have elderly care beds. With the health risks increase with age, the demand for medical services of the elderly becomes more prominent, generating more urgent needs for geriatric care. Geriatric care is mainly provided by secondary and tertiary specialized hospitals and geriatrics department of the general hospitals, undertaking diagnosis, surgery and inspection of intractable diseases for the aged population. For the large proportion of the elderly who needs palliative care at the end of life, Shanghai Municipal Government has launched a palliative care project, taking primary health care institutions as major pilot institutions. By establishing palliative care beds both in health institutions and at home, more palliative treatment and care services can be provided, and the life quality of dying patients can be improved. In addition, it has been demonstrated that preventive services like basic and major public health services for the elderly are cost-effective, such as physical examinations and screenings of colorectal cancer. Primary health care institutions serve as the main providers of preventive services and receive guidance from public health institutions.

In terms of service delivery, the old people are free to choose hospitals and primary health care institutions to receive medical services according to their needs. Institutionalized-care is primarily provided by nursing homes and elderly care institutions, given by professional caregivers. Home care, for instance, family beds are provided by medical staff from medical institutions. Every district in Shanghai carries out explorations in the delivery system of the elderly medical care, such as providing differentiated services based on need assessment and integrated health services, building a community level platform to promote the integration of pension service with medical service.

Overall, the functions of different levels of medical institutions in the pension and health care systems in Shanghai are relatively well-defined, providing corresponding range of services. Tertiary hospitals have a main function of therapeutic treatment, providing in-depth treatment of intractable diseases. It also has specialized departments of geriatrics, providing special medical care. Service areas of tertiary hospitals range from Shanghai to the whole Eastern China. Secondary hospitals are responsible for comprehensive health services of local residents and admitting patients transferring from primary health care institution and district hospitals. Referral patients include chronic disease patients with complications and chronic-to-acute disease patients. Community health care institutions are responsible for the "six in one" community health services, i. e. prevention, health protection, medical care, rehabilitation, health education and family planning service. They also undertake a large number of rehabilitation and nursing services, as well as chronic disease management and preventive services for the elderly. Meanwhile, it is encouraged to go to primary health institutions by the implementation of family doctor system. Under the guidance and support of the government, certain favorable policies have been made towards the medical services for the elderly. For instance, the project of standardized major public health service is launched at community level, containing health protection for the elderly people aged over 65, investigation of health risk factors, general physical examinations, disease prevention, self-care, injury prevention and self-saving; family doctor system is established, emphasizing contraction with elderly over 60 and long-term chronic prescription is implemented to solve the frequent treatment and repeated prescribing issue. Several community health centers begin to explore the "extended prescription", under which the prescriptions prescribed by big hospitals can be used further in the community, so that patients will be able to get the same medicine as large hospitals in the community, saving time and reducing the burden of costs.

2. Current status of Shanghai health financing system for the elderly

The health security system in Shanghai can be divided into four levels: backing, base layer, supplementary and voluntary layer. Backing is the medical assistance; base layer comprises two systems: the basic medical insurance for urban employees and basic medical insurance for urban and rural residents; supplementary layer comprises a community medical care mutual help program, CGT (General Confederation of Labor) worker's mutual aid security (WMAS), comprehensive help among residents in the community; voluntary layer includes voluntary purchased commercial life insurance and medical insurance.

Three basic medical insurance financing systems are the basic medical insurance for urban employees, basic medical insurance for urban and rural residents, and basic medical insurance for the land-requisitioned peasants. According to the retirement status and age, basic medical insurance for urban employees sets up a payment and security standard. For those of old age and have a long period of retirement, it hierarchically designs a lower deductible and a higher reimbursement rate. The practice of gradually increase the maximum payment cap benefits the elderly who have relatively high medical costs. When the self-paid accumulated medical expenses exceed a certain percentage of total annual income, it implements a medical insurance reduction tied to the annual income. Basic medical insurance for urban and rural residents also sets up a different financing and security standard according to age. In addition, there is an insurance of severe disease, focusing on the reduction of individual burden towards several severe diseases: uremia in hemodialysis, kidney transplant anti-rejection therapy, cancer treatment and some psychiatric disease treatment.

Supplementary medical insurance includes a community medical care mutual help program, CGT (General Confederation of Labor) worker's mutual aid security, comprehensive help among residents in the community, etc. Shanghai also sets up a medical assistance system, aiming to give reassurance to the low-income group. In terms of the elderly care, Shanghai Civil Affairs Bureau carries out the subsidy policy of pension service to the household elderly population aged over 60. Meanwhile, Shanghai Municipal Human Resources and Social Security Bureau (Health Insurance Office) establishes the health care program to give special subsidy to the insured aged over 70 in the basic medical insurance for urban employees. Regarding to the commercial health insurance, Shanghai establishes the health care plan of cancer prevention and individual severe disease protection.

Shanghai health security system has tilted toward the elderly population. For instance, according to the rules in the basic medical insurance for urban employees, retirees do not have to pay the insurance fee; In the basic medical insurance for urban and rural residents, the overall financing standard of elderly people aged 60 and over is higher than the standard for those under 60 years of age, whereas the individual contribution is approximately 70% to 50% of the population aged under 60. Among it, the individual contribution of those aged over 70 is less than that for the elderly above 60. Compared to the general population, the financing burden of the elderly is relatively small. A high level of reimbursement of medical expenses is mainly shown in the following aspects. Firstly, the elderly have a lower deductible. In the basic medical insurance for urban employees, the deductible of those aged 60 to 69 and over 70 who retired after January 1, 2001 is less than half of the staff's. For those who retired before December 31, 2000, the deductible is only 20% of the staff's. For retirees in the basic medical insurance for urban and rural residents, and basic medical insurance for the land-requisitioned peasants, their deductible is also only 40% of the staff's. Secondly, the elderly have a high reimbursement rate. The elderly reimbursement proportion when the medical expenses exceed the deductible is larger than that of the staff. There is a gradient payment, that is, the reimbursement rate of those who retired before December 31, 2000 is higher than the elderly aged 60 to 69 who retired after January 1, 2001, higher than the elderly aged over 70. In the supplementary medical insurance and medical assistance, there is also a special design for the elderly population and a specialized nursing care subsidy is established. For example, the community medical care mutual help program is specifically aimed at those who originally registered as a Shanghai household but is assigned to assist constructions and retired in other provinces, now reported as the Shanghai permanent residents. The Aged Foundation also gives out medical cards to the vulnerable elderly to help them seek for medical treatment.

3. Problems of the health service and financing system

First of all, the fragmentation of the management system leads to poor service convergence between institutions. Elderly population's medical service and nursing care are administrated by the department of health and civil affairs respectively, the criteria of hospitalization and discharge for the elderly hospitals and nursing homes is developed by the two different departments. Moreover, a unified need assessment system is in absence. Health insurance pays the patients according to the type of institutions, resulting in inequity in the use of health care service. That is, inadequacy as well as waste of resources coexist in the service delivery system for the old. For example, health insurances cover services in hospitals, resulting in the out-of-pocket payment in hospitals to be much lower than that at nursing homes or nursing at home. Thus, patients are unwilling to leave the hospitals. Meanwhile, the issue of medical care in nursing homes has not been solved. The aged population finds it difficult to obtain nursing care which meets their real need, which also affects the effective use of various kinds of elderly care service.

As for the allocation of health resources, Shanghai lacks a dominant high level gerontology center, and has insufficient nursing and rehabilitation resources. In terms of health personnel, there is a shortage of health needs evaluators, nurses and family doctors, leading to large amount of unmet service needs. In the health security system, it mainly emphasizes on the coverage of medical services, while neglecting of nursing and rehabilitation demand. The vast majority of nursing care programs are not covered by medical insurance. Since the long-term care insurance is not available at the present, the elderly have to bear the unaffordable burden of nursing fees, which negatively influences their nursing demands. In addition, the migrant elderly population is very large in Shanghai. Most of them have difficulty in transferring and renewing the medical insurance. They cannot use the health insurance in other provinces but have to pay out-of-pocket, resulting in a huge waste of resources.

With respect to health care utilization, waste and unreasonable utilization exist simultaneously. In Shanghai, the health care resources are relatively abundant, and all level institutions have explicit function positions. Although a series of policies have been introduced to encourage residents who have common and frequent disease to seek medical advice at the grassroots institutions, the elderly still prefer to go to large hospitals for medical treatment, leading to the low utilization of community health services. Due to the nature that elderly population is more likely to get sick and generate higher medical costs, it is difficult to control the overall expenses and implement regulations. Seen from the "$1+1+1$" contract data in 65 pilot communities, it has been calculated that the number of outpatient visit in 2016 is 20 times per capita. According to different age groups, the outpatient visit for the elderly aged over 70 and 80 reaches 50 times per capita, implying a problem of over-treatment. Nursing care resources are not adequate, however, in the process of service utilization, and the bed turnover rate is extremely low in nursing homes. Some elderly people enjoy the long-term care service in the geriatrics department of hospitals or elderly hospitals by using the existing health insurance.

4. Suggestions for the elderly health system

Firstly, the collaboration between departments should be improved to strengthen linkage mechanism. In response to the health needs of the elderly, a comprehensive service system should be established to improve the current fragmented situation. Shanghai has a good foundation of the family doctor system, health records and informationalization. It is recommended to further strengthen the communication between all levels of medical institutions to form a collaborative environment, to promote the collaboration between community health institutions, nursing homes and community elderly homes, and to develop the integration of pension service with medical service. On the other hand, long-term care needs assessment should be carried out. With different evaluation criteria dispersed in the departments of civil affairs, health and health insurance should be integrated to establish a unified municipal level need assessment system. Thus, it would be able to co-ordinate various kinds of health resources and the gradient security system can be improved. Connection channels between different services, i.e. hospitals, nursing homes and home care, should be established so that the elderly can get appropriate medical and nursing services.

Secondly, the health care delivery system for the elderly should be improved. To begin with, it is suggested to expand the total scale and to adjust the structure of health resources for the old. Specifically, it includes the establishment of a gerontology center to facilitate the construction and development of the subject of geriatrics in Shanghai, gradually reaching the leading position domestically and internationally. Shanghai tertiary hospitals are encouraged to develop the geriatrics subject, to promote geriatrics base construction, and to increase investments in the field of rehabilitation, general practice, nursing and other essential but weak subjects. Prevention and chronic disease management are to be strengthened, stepping up efforts to the construction of elderly care beds and training for related professionals. With the development of integrated health services, the family doctor system has been improved. Based on the core principle of continuing care, it is advised to focus on the integration between family, community and institutions in terms of elderly care, to provide an efficient institutional arrangement for the elderly. There is large emphasis on the optimal design of service programs to achieve integration. Take the family doctor contract system as an opportunity, the service boundary should be clarified and the incentive mechanism should be improved to further exert influence of family doctors on retaining medical costs. Thus, an expense management mechanism is to be established, taking contracted residents as the starting point and backed with the information systems. Finally, social capital is encouraged to participate in establishing pension institutions. The government, market and society should work together to promote a good pattern for the development of elderly health care.

Thirdly, the elderly health security system should be improved. The long-term care insurance system comes primarily in this aspect. It is recommended to top design and integrate all security policies of home-care, community-care and institution-care. Meanwhile, Shanghai should establish a multi-dimension long-term care insurance system which is insurance-based, supplemented by commercial insurance, and back up with social relief and welfare. This long-term care insurance is separated from but related to the basic health insurance. Afterwards, through the development of "targeted" burden reduction, it is advised to strengthen the protection of the elderly who suffer from serious illness. What's more, it is suggested to improve the remote reimbursement policy and encourage commercial insurance, making the personal accounts as the "bridge" between basic and commercial medical insurance.

Finally, the concept of "healthy aging" should be advocated for dissemination. Aging is a new modality instead of a disaster. The aging society in the future demonstrates that inevitably, implementation of policies requires consumption of resources, but it is a reasonable investment for the future society.

CHAPTER TWO   The Impact of Population Aging on Medical Expenses in Shanghai

Illness in the elderly is often chronic and involves co-morbidities. The elderly also have a greater probability of dying during the course of lives. Healthcare costs and utilization of healthcare services are closely related to health status, the disease spectrum, and medical needs. Healthcare costs and utilization of healthcare services are also closely associated with resource allocation and patterns of healthcare delivery.

1. The utilization and costs of medical service are higher among the elderly population whereby substantial resources may be wasted on the extreme elderly

The elderly have a higher morbidity rate compared to other age groups. Chronic diseases are a major component of the disease spectrum for older adults. The leading causes of hospitalization are cardiovascular disease, malignancies, and respiratory disease, and all three of these conditions require long-term care. **Healthcare needs should be paid attention to in the first place. Care for the elderly costs more and the elderly use more services than other age groups.** Healthcare needs are evident in two forms. **First, less than 20% of the population consumes nearly 50% of healthcare resources.** Individuals age 60 and over account for 19.5% of Shanghai's population but account for 52.2% of all outpatient and emergency visits, 45.3% of all hospital discharges, 63.2% of all emergency and outpatient costs, and 52.8% of all hospitalization costs. **Second, the costs of healthcare services per person per year need to be paid attention to. Services for the elderly cost about 6 times what services for other age groups cost.** On average, the elderly have 4.1 times the number of outpatient and emergency visits per person per year that children have and 4.5 times the number of outpatient and emergency visits that youths and adults have. Among the elderly, those aged 60~64 have 1.6 outpatient and emergency visits per person per month, and the average number of visits per person per year increases markedly with age. The elderly aged 80~84 have the largest number of outpatient and emergency visits, 3.8 visits per person per month. On average, the elderly have 3.0 times the number of admissions per year that children have and 3.5 times the number of admissions per year that youths and adults have. Total healthcare expenditures on the elderly are 6.3 times those on children and 5.7 times those on youths and adults.

Another key characteristic of the elderly is their high mortality rate. In the study of about 43 800 decedents in 2015, around 89.0% were 60 and over. Results of international studies have indicated that healthcare expenditures are affected by a proximity-to-death (PTD) phenomenon. Terminal patients are likely to use more healthcare resources, resulting in higher healthcare expenditures than expenditures on survivors (McGrail et al., 2000; Bartato et al., 2004; Polder et al., 2006; Blakey et al., 2014). **A PTD phenomenon is evident in Shanghai. With the proximity to death, the use of emergency and outpatient services and the costs of those services decrease while the use of inpatient services and the costs of those services abruptly increase (discussed in detail in point 5).**

Rising healthcare costs of the elderly and their increased utilization of services accord with general laws of nature. In Shanghai, healthcare expenditures on the elderly are about 6 times the healthcare expenditures on other age groups. A study by Reinhardt et al. (2003) indicated that medical costs for individuals aged 65 and over are more than 3 times the costs for individuals aged 34~44. A study by Lassman et al. (2014) revealed that the average medical costs per person for the elderly were 5 times the medical costs for children. A study by Hartman et al. (2008) found that the average medical costs per person for the elderly were more than 5.7 times the costs for youths and adults in the United States in 2004. **However, there has been a "rise" in the utilization of services by the extreme elderly and a "rise" in healthcare expenditures on the extreme elderly. The use and costs of**

healthcare in varieties of social characteristic elderly groups also present
significant difference, indicating that healthcare resources are being used
irrationally while ample room remains to rationally curtail healthcare
expenditures. One sign of the irrational use of healthcare resources is the
continual rise in the average healthcare expenditures per person for the extreme
elderly. Growing evidence from high-income countries has indicated that
healthcare expenditures in the elderly decrease markedly after age 70
(WHO, 2015). An analysis of expenditures and costs by the Torbay Care
Trust in the UK indicated that although the utilization of healthcare
services and the costs of those services generally increase with age but the
utilization of healthcare services and the costs of those services peak at ages
65 to 74. After those ages, expenditures on emergency admissions,
expenditures on non-urgent admissions, and inpatient and outpatient visits
decrease. This suggests that healthcare expenditures could be reduced in line
with demographic trends as the population ages. **The study by the Torbay
Care Trust stressed the importance of establishing an integrated system of
healthcare and long-term care in order to efficiently provide quality healthcare
services.** In contrast, the outpatient and emergency costs for the elderly in
Shanghai only began to decrease slightly at age 90 while hospitalization
costs continued to rise. The elderly aged 80 to 85 make 3.8 outpatient or
emergency visits per person per month, which corresponds to 1 visit per
week.

A second sign of the irrational use of healthcare resources is the relatively
high amount of healthcare expenditures on the elderly population in Shanghai
according to an analysis of Life Table Model. In Shanghai, the expected
healthcare expenditures over an individual's remaining lifetime after age 65
to 69 accounted for 69.0% of the expected healthcare expenditures over
their lifetime, and the expected healthcare expenditures over an
individual's remaining lifetime after ages 85 to 89 accounted for 27.0% of
the expected healthcare expenditures over their lifetime. For the elderly
who have lived past the age of 90, the medical costs until their death
account for 22.9% of their lifetime medical costs. The expected healthcare
expenditures over an individual's remaining lifetime after age 65 accounted
for 59.6% of the expected healthcare expenditures over their lifetime in

Michigan，the United States. The expected healthcare expenditures over an individual's remaining lifetime after age 85 accounted for 35.9% of the expected healthcare expenditures over their lifetime. Medical costs for the elderly population age 60 and older in Shanghai are higher than the medical costs in the United States which has the world's highest proportion of total healthcare expenditures to GDP.

2. The elderly population has specific healthcare needs and service model whereby the services provided by the healthcare facilities are fragmented

A key characteristic of geriatric diseases is the high incidence of co-morbidities, i.e. having two or more chronic diseases at the same time. Among the German elderly aged 70~85，24% of the elderly had 5 diseases. Among the Chinese elderly aged 70 and over，more than half suffers from multiple diseases（WHO，2015）. Among the population aged 60 and over in Shanghai，51.34% were seen for 4 or more diseases. A chronic disease requires long-term treatment and development of chronic disease management strategies to delay the progression of the disease and prevent disability. Co-morbidity must also be treated with a variety of drugs at the same time. **The model of healthcare services in Shanghai still focuses on the treatment of acute disease. Prevention needs to be enhanced as part of the healthcare service system, and chronic diseases of the elderly need to be effectively managed.** Public health facilities and facilities providing community healthcare services are the main organizations in Shanghai tasked with providing prevention and chronic disease management. According to calculations of healthcare expenditures（by facility），public health facilities in Shanghai accounted for 3.2% of healthcare costs in 2015，facilities providing community healthcare services accounted for 10.2%，and hospitals accounted for 71.7%.

In order to ensure the safe and effective treatment of disease，**numerous healthcare facilities and healthcare personnel should cooperate extensively, and technology and medicines should be used appropriately and collaboratively.** However，many elderly care confronted with inadequate coordination of healthcare services even in many developed countries. A survey conducted by Osborn et al. in 11 countries，including Britain，France，Germany，

Canada, and the United States, indicated that 40% to 50% of survey respondents had visited more than four physicians in a year. Issues cited by respondents included redundant examinations, conflicting information from different doctors, a lack of information shared among medical facilities, and a lack of uniformity in diagnosis and treatment. Like other provinces and cities in China, Shanghai uses a three-tier system of healthcare services. Facilities and personnel operate relatively independently, and the various types of facilities at different levels have not formed effective links, resulting in individual facilities that are highly efficient but a system that is inefficient. **The model of fragmented healthcare services needs to change, and the elderly need to receive unified, integrated healthcare services that span multiple specialties, multiple healthcare professions, and multiple facilities.** The current study was unable to track the exact number of physicians that a patient saw in a year. However, 19.76% of the elderly people aged 60 and over were hospitalized in 2 or more different medical facilities, and some elderly people were hospitalized in as many as 7 different facilities. 20.25% of the elderly received emergency or outpatient services at 2 or more different medical facilities, and some elderly people received services at as many as 8 different facilities.

The prevalence of disease among the elderly population is high, and so is the rate of disability. Medical services, medical care, and nursing care are needed. Currently, there is a shortage of resources and personnel in medical care and nursing care in Shanghai. The departments in charge of medical and nursing care are separate, and services are distinct from incentive policies. The degree of equitably and how efficiently nursing care is provided is greatly hampered. **First, there is a shortage of care resources.** The goal set by Shanghai is to have beds in care facilities for 1.5% of the elderly population aged 60 and over, with 0.75% of those beds in medical facilities. In 2015, there were 23,700 beds in nursing homes and facilities providing community healthcare services, so there is still a shortage of more than 10,000 beds to meet the target of 35,300 beds. **Second, care resources are both underutilized and wasted at the same time. A standard method of allocating and using resources based on need is lacking.** As an example, nursing homes are funded by health insurance premiums, so elderly residents of nursing homes can recoup their healthcare expenditures. A serious problem is that many elderly stay in nursing homes for longer than necessary while at-home care is seldom used since it is not covered by health insurance. **Disparate government, healthcare, and health insurance criteria for evaluation of medical and nursing needs need to be standardized, levels of medical and nursing care need to be clearly distinguished, and services need to be provided based on medical need. Different forms of services provided by hospitals, nursing homes, and home care need to be linked** to help the elderly obtain appropriate medical care and nursing care based on their health status.

3. With a higher proportion of elder patients to serve, primary care facilities need to be further improved

Primary care facilities (including community health service facilities, clinics and outpatient departments) and general practitioners serve as "gate keeper" of health management. Primary care services include (1) healthcare for the elderly, such as studies of health risk factors in the elderly aged 65 and over, physical examinations, and providing health instruction regarding the prevention of disease, self-care and injury prevention, and self-help; (2) since family doctor contract mechanism focuses on the elderly over age 60 and on patients with chronic disease, prescriptions are issued for longer periods so that patients with a chronic disease do not need to make frequent visits; and (3) some facilities have begun to explore issuing "extended prescriptions." "Extended prescriptions" from large hospitals can be filled at primary care facilities so that patients can avoid frequently going to a hospital to get a prescription filled. Moreover, some leverage has been applied in terms of health insurance premiums since primary care facilities receive a higher level of reimbursement than hospitals, in order to encourage the elderly to see physicians in the primary care facility first. Thus, primary care facilities are more attractive to the elderly than hospitals. 76.8% of the outpatient and emergency services of primary care facilities and 86.7% of their inpatient services are provided to the elderly.

Encouraging local patients to be seen by physicians in primary care facilities first is conductive to improving the efficient use of resources and

reducing medical expenditures. The per-visit fee from a primary care facility is lower than per-visit fee from a hospital (a hospital's fee for outpatient and emergency services is 2.4 times that of a primary care facility and a hospital's fee for inpatient services is 1.6 times that of a primary care facility). Relative to other age groups, the elderly go to primary care facilities and lower level hospitals more often than to higher level hospitals, and this helps to reduce medical expenditures. Expenditures of primary care facilities on emergency and outpatient services for the elderly are 9 times more than expenditures on children and 2 times more than expenditures on youths and adults. Expenditures of primary care facilities on inpatient services for the elderly are 9 times more than expenditures on youths and adults. Moreover, **patients at primary care facilities and lower level hospitals bear a lower percentage of costs, which can help reduce the medical burden of the elderly.** Patients at community health service facilities bear 9.9% of costs while patients at lower level hospitals such as long-term care hospitals bear 4.5% of costs. These percentages are much lower than the percentage of costs borne by patients at higher level hospitals (24.1%).

　　There is no doubt that encouraging local patients to be seen by physicians in primary care facilities first has greatly helped to improve the efficient use of healthcare resources in Shanghai. Although the elderly are seen by physicians in primary care facilities more than other age groups are, 50% or more of their outpatient or emergency visits and 90% or more of their inpatient services are in hospital. The use of health resources in Shanghai is an "inverted triangle," which is quite different from countries with healthcare systems that are performing well, such as the UK. Therefore, Shanghai still has a rough path to tread in terms of constructing additional primary care facilities and improving the quality of services. First, **the number of healthcare personnel and beds in primary care facilities need to be increased.** The current number of beds and the number of healthcare personnel in primary care facilities are both less than 15% of the total number. Second, **the capabilities of healthcare personnel need to be improved. Since primary care facilities mainly provide services to the elderly, healthcare personnel should receive enhanced training in chronic disease management and more focus on the needs of the elderly.** Healthcare personnel in primary care facilities have a lower level of education than healthcare personnel in hospitals. According to an old Chinese saying, "It takes ten years to grow trees but a hundred years to rear people". Enhancing the training of general practitioners, and improving their ability to provide comprehensive services for the elderly in particular, is a measure for both the immediate future and the long term. Finally, **hierarchical medical system needs to be promoted, health insurance premiums need to be increasingly leveraged, and a model of** "efficient" use of resources needs to be established. Order within the medical system has been disrupted since Shanghai implemented an "integration of medical card" in 2000. *Guiding Opinions on Promoting a Hierarchical Medical System* published by the Office of The State Council of China requires that a hierarchical medical system be established by 2017, and the system's capabilities should be comprehensively enhanced by 2020. However, a model that allows freedom to seek healthcare has great inertia, and changing this pattern of seeking healthcare in the short term will be difficult. Shanghai's "1+1+1" pilot program for residents to sign up with healthcare facilities allows residents to sign up with a community health service facility, a district-level hospital, and a municipal-level hospital where they will receive services first, and then get the policy benefits. The goal of this policy is to first start with Shanghai residents aged 60 and over and residents with chronic diseases. Through gradual changes, the program will bring most residents into the hierarchical medical system to create a scientific and rationally ordered way to seek healthcare. Among the first batch of 65 municipal-level pilot community health service facilities, 16 met basic requirements by the second quarter of 2015; 30 facilities were working to meet requirements and 19 facilities had not yet started. The data from a monitoring platform by August 2015 indicated that 40 pilot facilities had officially started the "1+1+1" signup program. More than 80,000 residents had signed up for the program. 77.57 percent of residents went to the healthcare facility they signed up with to receive outpatient services, and 64.45% went to the community health service facilities they signed up with. The next step is to further increase the signup rate and residents "compliance" with the facilities they selected. Moreover, the difference in insurance reimbursements for and the price of services provided by different levels of facilities needs to expand further in order to apply greater economic leverage to encourage residents to be seen by physicians in primary care facilities.

4. With specific population and disease bearing a greater burden of expenses, financing risks need to be spread out and long-term care insurance needs to be established

Within the framework of China's total expenditures on health, there are three main sources of financing (the government, the social sector, and the out-of-pocket payment). Roughly 60% of Shanghai's health financing comes from the social expenditure, which is the main source of financing, while 20% comes from government financing and 20% comes from out-of-pocket payment. The three systems of basic medical insurance account for about 85% of financing from the social expenditure. The system for collection of medical insurance premiums and payment of benefits greatly affects what medical costs are borne by patients. And the system has been designed with certain provisions for the elderly. **Compared to the general population, the elderly pay less in premiums.** As an example, the Urban Employee Basic Medical Insurance stipulates that retired people do not have to pay premiums for basic medical insurance. Under Urban and Rural Residents Basic Medical Insurance, the elderly aged $60 \sim 69$ and elderly aged 70 and over have a higher level of financing (70% and 50%, respectively) and lower premiums compared to people under age 60. **The elderly are reimbursed for a larger proportion of expenses, which results in the elderly bearing a lower percentage of costs.** As an example, the elderly bear 23.7% of hospitalization costs, which is 10.7 percentage points less than what youth and adult group bear. On one hand, the elderly have a low deductible that is $1/5 \sim 1/2$ of the deductible paid by youth and adult group; on the other hand, the elderly group is reimbursed for a larger percentage of expenses, and that percentage which is 5 percentage ~ 30 percentage points higher than what the youth and adult group is reimbursed for.

One problem is that **the level of financing and the level of reimbursement in the three schemes of basic medical insurance vary considerably. There is a large difference between the extent of services and the fee per visit, hence the** gap between the different systems of medical insurance needs to be narrowed further. The Urban Employee Basic Medical Insurance has the highest actual level of reimbursement, followed by the Urban Residents Basic Medical Insurance and then New Rural Cooperative Medical Insurance. The fee per visit covered by insurance systems for urban employee and residents is 8.1 times the fee covered by New Rural Cooperative Medical Insurance. After Urban Residents Basic Medical Insurance and New Rural Cooperative Medical Insurance were integrated in 2016, the gap between medical insurance for urban and rural residents disappeared. However, the disparity between the Urban Employee Basic Medical Insurance and the Urban and Rural Residents Basic Medical Insurance remains.

A second problem is that **some diseases incur more medical expenses, thus special attention needs to be paid to protection from financial risks**. According to a ranking of hospitalization costs for diseases among the elderly in Shanghai in 2015, the top three diseases were cardiovascular diseases, malignances, and respiratory diseases. The out-of-pocket payment per visit (patient co-payment + expenses beyond basic medical insurance coverage) ranged from 7,500~15,000 RMB, and the patient co-payment per visit ranged from 3,000~9,000 RMB. The three diseases mentioned have the highest prevalence and greatest impact on the elderly. The top three conditions requiring the largest co-payment are injury/poisoning (18,700 RMB), malignancies (14,900 RMB), and musculoskeletal disorders (12,900 RMB). The out-of-pocket payments for these conditions are also high, ranging from 6,000~9,000 RMB. Therefore, the Urban Employee Basic Medical Insurance has established a system to alleviate the overall burden on patients and meanwhile the Urban Residents Basic Medical Insurance features catastrophic illness insurance to reduce the medical expenses borne by patients with a catastrophic illness. **Catastrophic insurance covers dialysis for severe uremia, anti-rejection therapy after a kidney transplant, treatment of malignancies, and treatment of some psychiatric illnesses. The diseases covered are limited. For instance, cardiovascular disease with highest prevalence among the elderly and highest hospitalization costs is not covered. In principle, the scope of covered diseases needs to be expanded in accordance with prevalence, the course of the disease, and its costs.**

The third problem is that **the medical insurance system in Shanghai places considerable emphasis on coverage of medical services while neglecting nursing care and rehabilitation needs. Long-term care insurance needs to be promptly implemented.** Nursing care and rehabilitation needs of the elderly population and terminal patients markedly increased, but most nursing care and rehabilitation is not covered by medical insurance. On one hand, the lack of long-term care insurance has suppressed rational medical needs; on the other hand, some patients who only need nursing care choose to be seen by hospitals for financial reasons. As mentioned earlier, most expenses for facilities providing community healthcare services and care facilities for the elderly are covered by medical insurance while the elderly living at home or in a nursing home do not receive social insurance benefits, leading to bed vacancies.

5. With end-of-life hospitalization costs increasing dramatically, the resource allocation needs to be optimized and costs need to be rationonalized in line with the characteristics of care

During the last 2 years before death, healthcare service utilization and healthcare spending of the elderly population increase markedly. The healthcare facilities and resources used in the 2 years before death change as well. **Inpatient services and costs of hospitalization increase significantly at the end of life.** The average emergency and outpatient costs per decedent in tertiary hospitals are 1.5 times the costs for the entire population (including survivors and decedents). The average emergency and outpatient costs per decedent in primary and secondary hospitals are 1.4 times the costs for the entire population. The average emergency and outpatient costs per decedent in community health centers are 76.28% of the costs for the entire population. Costs of hospitalizing a terminal elderly patient in a tertiary hospital are 15 times the costs of hospitalization for the entire population. Costs of hospitalizing a terminal elderly patient in a primary or secondary hospital are 16 times the costs of hospitalization for the entire population. While among the elderly population aged 60 and over, costs of hospitalizing a terminal elderly patient in a community health center are 64 times the costs of hospitalization for the entire population. In the 2 years before death，each elderly decedent is hospitalized averagely once every 6 months，which is 19 times more often than the entire elderly population is hospitalized，regardless of proximity to death. The average hospitalization costs per elderly decedent have increased as much as $7.3 \sim$ fold (40,000 RMB)，compared to costs for the entire elderly population. **Primary care facilities account for a larger share of care provided at the end of life.** Seventy percent of emergency and outpatient visits by terminal elderly patients are to community health centers，while the proportion of inpatient services for terminal elderly patients provided at primary level is 7% (in the entire elderly population the number is below 5%). These figures indicate that **patients are more likely to go to community health institutions for health services at the end of their lives. However, the limited number of beds at community level (17,000 beds, accounting for 14% of the total) and prolonged stays may mean that the healthcare needs of terminal patients are not being met.** Gozalo et al. (2015) found that some healthcare costs may be replaced by other costs. An increase in hospice use was associated with significant decreases in the rates of hospital transfers (2.4 percentage-point reduction) and intensive care unit (ICU) use (7.1 percentage-point reduction). According to Hartman et al. (2008)，per person spending for those aged 85 and over fell from 6.9 times higher than that of the working-age population in 1987 to just 5.7 times higher in 2004，which is almost entirely attributable to a low rate of growth in nursing home care (nursing home care accounts for the largest share of all health spending for the population age 85 and older). In Shanghai，the average emergency and outpatient costs per person in community health institutions were 1/3 of the costs in tertiary hospitals and hospitalization costs in community health institutions were 1/2 of the costs in tertiary hospitals. Allocating additional resources to primary care and encouraging patients to be seen at primary care facilities are key ways to use funds more efficiently，but end-of-life care is still predominantly provided by hospitals. **Healthcare resources at the level of primary care, and particularly nursing and hospice resources need to be enhanced so that healthcare needs at the end of life can be met and healthcare costs can be curtailed.**

The widespread controversy surrounding the relationship between age and healthcare spending is largely due to the "inconvenient fact" that a PTD phenomenon occurs. Results of the current study indicate that hospitalization costs incurred in the last month before death account for approximately 30% of the cumulative hospitalization costs incurred in the 2 years prior to death. The average daily hospitalization costs are increased by 50% from 24 months before death to 1 month prior to death, indicating the occurrence of a PTD phenomenon. However, this finding does not conflict with the pressure that aging places on healthcare financing. The occurrence of a PTD phenomenon further reveals how aging causes an increase in healthcare spending. A PTD phenomenon is not merely the result of age and health status but it is also a result of changes in end-of-life care and patterns of seeking healthcare. The combined effect of age and population size (caused by increased life expectancy) has resulted in a larger number of people with vast medical needs, challenging the sustainability of the healthcare service and financing system. In order to better meet the needs of patients, excessive medical costs at the end of life should be be rationally curtailed and more attention should be paid to the population with a heavier disease burden.

To control waste, the relationship between medical services and ethical issues needs to be properly addressed, and patients with high medical costs, frequent outpatient and emergency visits, frequent hospitalizations, and prolonged stays should be monitored. **Firstly, high medical costs need to be monitored, and the rationality and value of medical services should be assessed.** End-of-life medical costs for 16% of the decedents in the current study exceeded 150,000 RMB, total medical costs of which accounted for half of all medical costs for the patients studied. Medical costs were as high as 4.06 million RMB. Medical costs for the top 1% of the decedents (approximately 500 patients) amounted to 416 million RMB (with an average of 830,000 RMB per decedent), while medical costs for the top 5% of terminal patients (approximately 2500 patients) amounted to 1.085 billion RMB (with an average of 430,000 RMB per decedent). **Secondly, prolonged stays and frequent emergency and outpatient visits should be monitored and unnecessary medical treatments should be prevented by appropriate referral and redirection.** Results of regression analysis indicated that the duration of hospitalization is a key factor influencing hospitalization costs[①]. Because of medical costs in closer proximity to death, several patients spent the whole year in hospital, seeing it as a nursing home.

Among those patients who were hospitalized for over 180 days, 50.11% were hospitalized in community health centers, 21.29% resided in nursing homes, 5.63% were hospitalized in mental hospitals, and over 16% were hospitalized in a general hospital or TCM hospital. These patients should be monitored so that those with actual medical needs can be transferred to primary health institutions or receive at-home care. Patients with an incurable condition or who will not benefit from treatment should not be hospitalized for a prolonged period, either [②]. In the 2 years before death, elderly patients made as many as 471 cumulative outpatient visits, meaning that patients were seen by healthcare facilities about 20 times each month (approximately 1 visit each workday). This is clearly irrational representing a serious waste of medical resources. Over 10% of the elderly population made more than 65 visits to the outpatient or emergency department at the end of their lives while 5% made over 92 visits.

An analysis of data related to the utilization of medical services by the elderly, the costs of those services, and end-of-life care in Shanghai yielded several findings. The elderly have a higher morbidity rate compared to other age groups, chronic diseases are a major component of diseases affecting the elderly, the elderly have a high incidence of co morbidities, the elderly frequently use medical services, and care for the elderly is expensive. The finding that the elderly use several times more medical resources than other age groups is consistent with accounts overseas. However, there has been a "rise" in the utilization and costs by the extreme elderly indicating that medical resources are not being used rationally. Numerous healthcare facilities and healthcare personnel should cooperate extensively, technology and medicines should be used appropriately and

---

① Wu H, Wang C, Guo H. Analysis of several factors influencing hospitalization costs, Chinese Journal of Hospital Statistics, 2004, 11(2): 138—139.

② Luo R. Analysis of inpatients with medical insurance costs over 100,000 RMB [J]. Chinese Health Resources, 2005(6): 41—42.

collaboratively to cope with the high morbidity rate of elderly. In Shanghai, the overall number of primary care facilities needs to increase and the capabilities of healthcare personnel need to improve. Under the three-tier system of healthcare services, facilities and personnel operate relatively independently, and the various types of facilities at different levels have not formed effective links, resulting in individual facilities that are highly efficient but a system that is inefficient. While the 13th Five-year Plan is in effect, efforts need to focus on improving the quantity and quality of primary care and the model of fragmented healthcare services needs to change so that the elderly receive integrated, unified healthcare services that span multiple specialties, multiple healthcare professions, and multiple facilities. The UK's experience indicates that medical costs increase with age, but those costs peak at ages 65 to 74. After those ages, expenditures on emergency admissions and non-urgent admissions, and inpatient and outpatient visits decrease. The researchers believe that this benefits from the establishment of an integrated system of healthcare and long-term care, which will provide the health care service with higher efficiency and quality. Equitability of care is an issue in China since the level of financing and reimbursement in the three systems of basic medical insurance vary considerably. There is a large difference between the extent of services and the fee per visit, so the gap between different systems of medical insurance needs to be narrowed further. Some diseases incur more medical expenses, but catastrophic illness insurance has been established. However, the diseases covered are limited. As an example, cardiovascular disease is most prevalent among the elderly and incurs the largest hospitalization costs but is not covered. In addition, special attention needs to be paid to protection from financial risks. A system to cap the out-of-pocket payment should be promptly created. High medical costs need to be monitored, the rationality and value of medical services should be assessed, and patients with prolonged stays should be appropriately referred and redirected to other facilities. Moreover, Shanghai's medical insurance system has placed great emphasis on coverage of medical services while neglecting nursing care and rehabilitation needs. Long-term care insurance needs to be promptly implemented.

The next step is to compare Shanghai and the UK in terms of the utilization of medical services by the elderly and the costs of those services, to ascertain differences, and to analyze the reasons for differences in resource allocation, the reasons for different models of healthcare services, and the reasons for different incentives. In November 2016, the Shanghai team traveled to London to conduct an on-site study. Results of that study revealed aspects that Shanghai can learn from, such as emphasizing the system of general practitioners and health management, adhering to an efficient model of resource utilization that is oriented toward primary care and prevention, implementing an integrated model of healthcare, and conducting personnel training. These aspects will be reviewed and summarized in stage Ⅲ, and models will be developed to simulate and predict the potential benefits of changes in phase Ⅳ.

CHAPTER THREE　Ten Strategies to Cope with the Aging Society

1. Face up to aging challenge: financial challenge

The healthcare financing policy must be aligned with the final objectives of universal health coverage of aging population: to ensure everyone to access necessary healthcare service (e. g: disease prevention, health promotion, disease treatment and rehabilitation therapy) without financial problem[1]. According to Shanghai Academy of Social Science (SASS)[2], the total population of Shanghai will show a sustained growth, with a total population of 26.50 million expected in 2020, continuing to rise until 2035 (28.72 million) and falling after, to 27.83 million in 2050. While the aging trend continues, it is expected that the proportion of elderly people aged 60 years and over will reach 21.5% in 2020 and 44.8% in 2050. In correspondence with that, this study combined per capita health expenditure trends from 2010 to 2015 to predict medical expenses. Resident

---

[1]　World health report 2010. Health systems financing: The path to universal coverage. Geneva: World Health Organization; 2010 (http: //www. who. int/whr/2010/en/).

[2]　Zhou, H W. Forecast of Shanghai population development based on Multi-factor Population Parameter Hypothesis.

population's medical expenses increase year by year, rising from 107. 2 billion RMB in 2015 to 186.18 billion RMB in 2020. In 2050 it is expected to reach 884. 15 billion RMB. The proportion of medical expenses for the elderly over 60 will increase from 54.4% in 2015 to 58.0% in 2020, and 80.8% in 2050. The growth of large medical costs for aging population requires the need to build sustainable health financing systems.

1.1　Expand financing channels and optimize the structure

At present, the medical security system of the elderly in Shanghai is relatively fragmented in structure, which leads to unfairness of different social groups, brings remarkable difference in security benefits, and ineffective management of security systems. It is proposed to design through top-level, expand financing channels, and to build a healthy aging system which is based on social insurance and commercial insurance as a supplement, whilst put social relief and welfare as a floor to the system, and to integrate the security policies of home care, community care and institution care.

1.1.1　Expand diversified financing channels of medical insurance. Different age and different levels of economic groups require different level of healthcare services. Although most residents are covered by basic medical insurance, the burden of expense between different security systems remains. Combining with insured population and fund operation status, it is found that in the group of Urban Residents Basic Medical Insurance (URBMI) and New Rural Cooperative Medical Insurance (NRCMI), elderly is in a high proportion of all the insured, while in the Urban Employee Basic Medical Insurance (UEBMI), personal medical saving account balance is more concentrated in younger people. At current stage, in the market of commercial insurance to aging population, there are limited products and little volume. It is possible to explore a co-develop way that combining the basic insurance and commercial insurance, for example, improving the personal medical saving account functions of workers by encouraging the purchase of commercial health insurance. In December 2016, the Shanghai Government issued the Notice on the "Voluntary use of accumulated surplus fund in Medical Saving Accounts to Purchase Commercial Insurance", which clearly stipulated that the personnel who is insured by UEBMI can use the accumulated surplus in their medical saving account to purchase specific commercial insurance products that is approved by CIRC (China Insurance Regulatory Commission) and endorsed by Shanghai government for themselves in accordance with voluntary principle. Shanghai Insurance Industry has correspondently developed two exclusive commercial insurance products which are "low premium, high security": one covers out-of-pocket in-hospital expenditure, the first personal health insurance product in this country that covers out-of-pocket in-hospital expenditure of elders. The reimburse rate on reasonable and necessary out-of-pocket expenses is 50%. The other one is an improved dread disease insurance, which expands the scope of the disease while with substantial lower premium than current products in market[①]. The implementation of this policy benefits many parties. For the government, it helps with sustainable development of basic health insurance system for urban workers and improves the efficiency of medical saving accounts. For the insurance industry, it helps to further expand the coverage of commercial insurance thus enable them to play a role in the multi-level medical security system. And for those who are protected, it is a good solution to their heavy burden caused by out-of-pocket expense and dread diseases, to protect them from the poverty brought by disease.

1.1.2 Develop long-term care insurances. With a deeper aging of population, elders require more nursing care services, thus the burden of nursing services are also gradually increasing. Establishment of the long-term care insurance can be beneficial in many aspects: It is conducive to the protection of the basic rights and interests of disabled people to enhance their decent and dignified life quality, and promote the traditional Chinese culture and virtue. It is also helpful to improving people's well-being, promoting social justice and maintaining social stability. In December 2016, the Shanghai Municipal Government issued the "Shanghai long-term care insurance pilot approach". During the two-year pilot period, it will provide long-term care insurance for the insured people who have been

---

① Shanghai: Purchasing commercial health insurance by medical saving accounts next year. http://business.sohu.com/20161227/n477100888.shtml

assessed and rated at level 2 to 6 in their validity period. The services include community and home care, nursing care, hospital care and so on. For different levels of care services there are different payment ratios, which can guide an ordered care service. At this stage, this insurance covers all the insured people of the UEBMI and elders of 60 and above of URBMI. The financing of long-term care insurance for UEBMI is from employer, accounting 1% of average payment base, for elders of URBMI, individual need to pay 15% of the premium. However, with the gradual advancement of long-term care insurance, it is necessary to take population structure, medical expenses, nursing costs, industry development and other factors into account, with the base of economic and social development, as well as the actual fund operation, to consider about the combined impact and set a dynamic multi-channel financing mechanism.

1.2 Construct incentive and restraint mechanisms to ensure financing efficiency

The financing policy should guarantee a series of systematic incentives to promote integrated health services, rather than encourage individual events isolated to make a temporary reaction[①]. To be more specific, the fund service efficiency can be improved by optimizing resources from both suppliers and demander side.

From the side of demander, it is suggested to play the guiding role of insurance. Regarding to elders' common and frequent disease, the gaps of reimbursement ratio in different hospital levels can be expanded to guide an orderly medical-seeking pattern. This must base on an extensive HTA (health technology assessment) and economic analysis on policy intervention. Economic incentives should be offered to preventive measures and long-term care (including rehabilitation, palliative care and end of life care) which delay or prevent elders' function declining.

From the side of supplier, not only the compensation of medical staff needs to be increased, but the incentives to staffs in those community or primary care agencies which provide prevention, chronic disease management,

---

① World report on ageing and health. 2015. http: //www. who. int /ageing / publications/world-report-2015/en/.

and rehabilitation services should also be guaranteed. In the meanwhile，the healthcare service system must be rationalized，in combine with other measures like payment system reform. For example，according to the "1+ 1＋1" medical union pilot policy，which is already implemented in Shanghai，global budget can be implemented in medical union，and the general practitioners can be paid by capitation. By defining a clear medical services list and payment standard in each healthcare provider at different level，their capability of carrying out expected services is enhanced. The policy interpretation and promotion strategy need to be developed carefully[①].

2. Service model transformation: develop the integrated care model for the elderly

With the improvement of health of residents in Shanghai，the average life expectancy is increasing while the disease and death spectrum are gradually changing. Traditional healthcare model，which is called "disease-centered"，is now being replaced by the "people-centered" biological-psychological-social healthcare model. The elderly people's demand on healthcare services is increasingly diversified，which requires policy makers to develop an elderly centered，integrated care model based on their characteristics.

2.1 Elderly-oriented service

It is found that among the elderly in shanghai，the prevalence of chronic disease and co-morbidity is high. The number of patients who go to doctor for four or more than four diseases is about half of the whole. Chronic disease requires long-term，regular treatment while co-morbidity requires multi-pronged treatment. In addition，rehabilitation service should be provided，to prevent and postpone any physical or mental disability due to disease. At present，the health service model of the elderly in Shanghai is still mainly focused on treatment to acute diseases，and treatments often occur in multiple healthcare institutions，which lead to records incoherence

---

　① World Bank Group, WHO and 3 Chinese ministries. Healthy China: Deepening health reform in China building high-quality and value-based service delivery. 2016. http: //www. wpro. who. int/china/publications/health-reform-in-china.pdf.

and service fragmentation. Learning from the UK experience, a new elderly-centered service model can be established by stages, following the three aspects: (1) **Resources are gradually transferred to community and health promotion.** It is adviced to restrict the size of public hospitals, control the number of hospital beds, put more manpower and resource into community health care and focus more on behavior and life style intervention. It is important to improve residents' understanding to health, and reduce or eliminate the risk factors that affect health. (2) **Services are provided based on demands.** Experience of UK integrated care pathway can be adopted for reference. The key point is to first screen out the focus diseases and groups (such as older elderly population), then identify their priorities through a comprehensive assessment on physical status, family support and so on. Thirdly, to establish a series of standardized integrated care pathways, including diagnostic criteria, service standards, referral standards, prevention services packages, etc. (3) **Personalized service programme is developed.** It is suggested to formulate the service package which is targeted and personalized to the elderly. A permanent multidisciplinary service team is responsible for providing services and conducting health management.

2.2 Integrated service model

Integrated service model is not only based on the community, but also the consideration of overall healthcare system. The form of integration can be divided into the following levels. (1) **Horizontal.** Horizontal integration includes communication and cooperation among elderly service institutions including hospitals, nursing homes and aged care facilities, as well as organic combination of services such as health care, social services and so on. Joint meeting mechanism can be set up between health, civil affairs, medical insurance sectors, disabled persons' federation and other government agencies, with a management team to coordinate with related affairs. (2) **Vertical.** Vertical integration refers to optimizing the tiered medical services by consolidating the function positioning of medical institutions of each level and the "gatekeeper" system. First-treatment in community and two-way referrals are to be achieved step by step by a series of preferential policies and services including long prescription, health management, referral priority, tertiary hospital experts visits, and extending the prescription, in order to ensure the continuity on the services of prevention, diagnosis, treatment, rehabilitation, functional recovery and the improvement of mobility. The pilot program "$1+1+1$" in Shanghai is a good sample of exploration in this way. (3) **Within institutions. Integration within institutions** includes accelerating the delivery of training program to professionals in primary healthcare institutions, such as traditional Chinese medicine practitioners, community nurses, rehabilitation therapists, nutritionists, psychological counselors and social workers. Team construction of multidisciplinary service needs to be strengthened with the general practitioner as the core. In large comprehensive hospitals, multidisciplinary experts can provide disease consultation and integrated treatment service to elderly patients. (4) **Prevention and treatment service. Service** delivery should be transferred from disease-oriented to the prevention and treatment combination, together with attention to social and psychological factors. The community health center is the foundation to carry out comprehensive, continuous and specific health management to elders. Furthermore, mental diseases caused by separated living, empty-nest family and social pressure are important influencing factors of the elderly people's health status, which requires more attention on prevention and disease controlling. (5) **Physicians and patients.** As learned from the UK experience, patient involvement and independence is critical. From the view of suppliers, service providers should participate in the implement of policies on physician signing-up, tiered medical service and community general practitioner, to encourage the elderly to participate in health management and medical decision-making, therefore the trust between physicians and patients can be built. From the view of consumers, health education and public awareness should be strengthened, proper health knowledge from formal channels should be provided, to encourage patients to take more responsibility for their own health.

An integrated service can be more efficient in terms of resource utilization and health improvement. Thus an effective way to address challenges of aging population is to set an elderly-centered, integrated care model, to build multidisciplinary service team that focuses on general practitioners, to explore personalized service plan and to promote the integration of health service and social service.

3. Resource planning: emphasize on coordination, integration and optimization

While the population aging in Shanghai has become increasingly prominent, the nursing issue of the elderly is becoming more and more conspicuous and the supply of service has become a key factor restricting the development of elderly care.[①]

This is reflected in the following three aspects: **the first is the significant shortage**[②] of ward beds, healthcare and nursing professionals, which can hardly meet the demand. **The second is the uneven quality.** Some agencies are in poor facility and their professionals are suffering from poor education and high turnover rate. **The third is misallocation of resources.** In Shanghai, the resource and quality distribution between different districts and agencies is unequal. Vacant and deficient of ward bed exist at the same time. Both home-based nursing and agency nursing are in lack of medical support.[③] To get rid of these three constraints, we need to use multipronged approaches from several aspects.

3.1　In terms of planning, commit the elderly service resource planning based on big data

Shanghai has formulated the "Special Plan for the Layout of Elderly Care Facilities in Shanghai (2013-2020)", "Shanghai Elderly Medical Care Service System Planning (2016-2020)", emphasizing that the provision of old-age care service resources should be increased. The first thing is to build a big data network according to social demographic profile and the distribution of healthcare, nursing and community service agencies within

---

① Zhang Q, Gao X D. Analyzing the long-term care needs of the elderly population and its factors: Based on Shanghai survey data analysis[J]. Northwest population, 2016 (2): 87—90.

② Ding H S, Du L X, Zhao W, et al. On the demands, expenses and problems of elderly care in Shanghai[J]. Scientific Research on Aging, 2014(2): 47—53.

③ Jiao X, Hou J L, Tian Z P. Research on the supply and demand estimation of aged care and the establishment of long-term care system in Shanghai [J]. Chinese Hospital Management, 2014, 34(7).

the region. The second thing is, based on the data network, to co-ordinate with regional healthcare, nursing, rehabilitation and other resources, the government should incorporate the integration of elderly services into the regional function planning and construction. In the meanwhile, we must commit to a scientific resource planning process and encourage the development of regional integration and expansion of resources to fully mobilize and use the in-stock and incremental resources, and also to adjust the structure of various types of institutions at all levels for the elders to provide diversified, comprehensive and systematic service.

3.2　In terms of funding, accelerate the overall resource planning through long-term nursing insurance

The initial batch of long-term nursing insurance in the country launches in 15 pilot cities including Shanghai. In January 2017, Shanghai carried out its pilot projects in 3 districts, which are Xuhui, Putuo and Jinshan.① **In terms of suppliers,** any healthcare, nursing and social services provided by a certified agency, regardless of healthcare agency, nursing agency or home-nursing agency, will be enrolled in coverage scope of insurance. **The long-term nursing insurance breaks the barrier between different sectors that hold accountable for healthcare and pension services, and put the social insurance fund in a big picture.** While the pilot progresses, the project will further expand the list of services. **In terms of demanders,** long-term nursing insurance enhances their purchasing power of elderly care services. On the one hand, it stimulates the market to attract all kinds of business entities to participate in equal and sharing funds. On the other hand, the dynamic market will provide a wide range of services, to fully meet the needs of different levels.

3.3　In terms of agency, promote integration between healthcare and nursing agencies through various approaches

The approaches of integration include: **1) medical sector in pension agency.** The Shanghai government has added"50 New Medical Sector in Old-

---

① Shanghai Municipal Government. Shanghai long-term care insurance pilot measure. http://www.shanghai.gov.cn/nw2/nw2314/nw2319/nw12344/u26aw51124. html[2016-12-29].

age Institutions" into the municipal government practical projects in 2015 and 2016. The Ministry of Health actively guided all eligible agencies to establish medical sectors and issued "Guidance for Shanghai pension agencies to set up medical sector". **2) pension sector in healthcare agency.** The Ministry of Health encourages healthcare agencies to host or set up pension institutions, which is entitled to a ward bed subsidy and monthly operating subsidy from civil administration sector. **3) cooperation between healthcare and pension agencies.** One possible approach is the cooperation between community healthcare service center and pension agency. Shanghai has developed "The Standard of Contract-based Services between Community Health Service Centers and Pension Agencies", and actively facilitated the community health service centers and pension service agencies to establish a contract-based cooperation service model. By the end of 2015, 100% of all pension agencies had been contracted. **Another way is the cooperation between community and medical institutions.** In existing community care institutions like care center and other service center, social workers and volunteers from healthcare center or nursing station can provide door-to-door service. By the end of 2016, 64% of community foster agencies had signed a contract with a medical institution, and this rate is expected to reach 100% by the end of 2017. **4) use the community platform to integrate all elderly service resources.** Among 141 basic services under 16 categories that are provided by the Community Health Service Center, 69 have put elderly population as focus. Community care, home care, health management and relieving services represent 57% of the total workload.

We also encourage some of the tertiary and secondary hospitals to transform to elderly nursing home and encourage ward bed conversion in comprehensive hospitals. District comprehensive hospital that provides elderly care beds can be granted a one-time subsidy of 10,000 RMB per bed through the social welfare fund. In additional to that, social forces can be mobilized to participant in social pension services, with particular emphasis on the elderly population with low income, older age, physical or mental disability, etc. This includes the encouragement and support to social forces to set up elderly service agencies, as well as voluntary and charitable organizations to implement various elderly care activities.

3.4   In terms of personnel, build a talent pool of practitioners

For now, China has not yet formed a standardized occupational access, training and evaluation system for the elderly caregivers, resulting in the irregularity of the talent team. The elderly population has a large and increasing demand on nursing services, which needs an accelerated construction of professional team from the view of resource planning: **(1) Develop vocational category for caregivers.** The China Nursing Career Development Plan (2016-2020) has mentioned that "to speed up the team construction of nursing professionals". The government should explore a way to integrate elderly care workers, hospital works and housekeeping personal into one team and issue same professional certificate of "Elderly Nursing Worker" at national or local level. **(2) Establish a way to develop nursing professionals.** The first thing is to produce a serious of guidance documents on the standard of participating, education, evaluation, etc. And the second is to improve the training, certifying and on-boarding system for nursing professionals. The duration and content of training can differ from different practice or responsibilities. The third thing is, to optimize the continuous education that can update their certificate regularly and encourage junior professionals to obtain a higher-level certificate by attending training and examination. **(3) Improve the remuneration of nursing staffs.** This means to establish a nursing professional team with moderate scale and good structure. The higher level the professionals are, the higher income they receive.

An advisable resource allocation would not be achieved overnight, and the solid implementation and improvement of planning, practicing, evaluation at all aspects are essential. Shanghai has made a number of meaningful explorations in the integration of medical care. We need to keep our advantages on scientific planning and top-level designing, emphasize the co-ordination, integration and optimization of existing resources, and actively and steadily promote the implementation of all measures.

4. Proper utilization of healthcare services: control the cost in effective ways

China has entered into an aged society while its economy has not yet developed, which is known as "Getting old before getting rich". Medical costs have increased sharply as the number of older people grows, and the income balance of the medical insurance fund has been severely challenged as a result of the reduction in labor force. Elderly people suffer from multiple diseases and high medicine costs. There exist difficulties in cost control and in regulation as well.

4.1 Monitoring on irrational use of healthcare services

In terms of controlling waste, efforts must be taken to monitor people with high medical costs, excess visiting time, increased hospitalization time and prolonged hospital days. It was found that in 2015, the comparative consumption of medical resource between the elderly population and other age groups was aligned with general experience worldwide. However, for older elderly, there are "up tails" in both service utilization and medical costs. The results of Life Table Model analysis show the relatively high medical expenses among the elderly population in Shanghai, suggesting irrational use of medical resources. Among the patients in the terminal stage, 16% of them generated more than RMB 150,000 medical expenses in the last 2 years of life, accounting for half of the total expenses of the sample population. The maximum medical expense was RMB 4.05 million. Medical costs for the top 1% of the patients in terminal stage (approximately 500 patients) amounted to RMB 416 million (with an average of RMB 830,000 per capita), while medical costs for the top 5% of terminal patients (approximately 2,500 patients) amounted to RMB 1.085 billion (with an average of RMB 430,000 per capita). The results of the regression analysis showed that the length of stay was one of the main influencing factors of hospitalization expenses.[1] Among all cases in this survey, the longest length of stay reached a whole year. In this case, hospital was turned into a nursing home. Among the patients whose length of a hospital-stay exceeded 180 days, 50.11% were hospitalized in community health service centers, 21.29% in nursing houses, and 5.63% in psychiatric hospitals. However, more than 16% of them were still

---

① Wu H Y, Wang C Y, Guo H X. Analysis of factors influenced by hospitalization expenses[J]. Chinese Journal of Hospital Statistics, 2004 11(2): 138—139.

hospitalized in general hospitals and TCM hospitals. Here are some proposals to address these issues:

4.1.1　Monitor high medical expenses and assess the rationality and value of health services. Independent medical expense censor mechanisms in several countries can be adapted. Japan and South Korea both set up independent medical expense censorship with examiners from insurance agencies, physicians and patients representatives, to review medical expenses among all healthcare institutions, ages and diseases[1][2]. In Taiwan, the expenses are reviewed by the health insurance agency. There are also technical reviews on sample cases in additional to the general cost review, for instance, the correctness of disease diagnosis, the necessity of medical testing and examination, the consistency between treatment or surgery and diagnosis, compliance of the type and dose of medication[3].

4.1.2　Monitor the length of long-term hospitalization and the number of outpatient and emergency visits, and prevent waste by rational referral and redirection. Patients with actual medical needs can be transferred to primary health institutions or receive at-home care. Patients with an incurable condition or who will not benefit from treatment should not be hospitalized for a prolonged period, either[4]. In the 2 years before death, elderly patients made as many as 471 cumulative outpatient visits, meaning that patients were seen by healthcare facilities about 20 times each month. And 77 patients seek outpatient services for more than 200 times, suggesting severe waste of medical services that need in-depth investigation.

4.1.3　Reinforce the supervision over healthcare agencies. The reimbursement rate of Shanghai medical insurance schemes is relatively high. However, the data showed that among all OOP in the inpatient department, around 60% are copayment and 40% are beyond reimbursement range. Among these

---

① Zhai S G. The overview of national health insurance expense payment system in Korea [J]. China Health Insurance,2012(7): 70—72.

② Lv XJ. Medical point payment in Japan[J]. China Health Insurance,2010(6): 58—59.

③ Ding H S, Du L X, Li F, et al. Lump-sum prepayment of health insurance in Taiwan [R],2012.

④ Luo R X,Medical expenses analysis on the hospitalization cases of more than ten thousand yuan of medical insurance [J]. China Health Insurance,2005(6): 41—42.

service items beyond reimbursement range, those with a positive cost-effective result and equivalent to social-economic development status should be included into the scope of reimbursement. Other out-of-pocket items should be monitored and emphasis should be put on the elderly population and on key diseases. Big data technology could be applied to monitor the overall out-of-pocket expenses in all agencies and the results should be made public.

4.2　Reduce expenses through the transformation of healthcare service model

The service model in Shanghai is disease-oriented, and emergency-treatment dominated. Modern Medicine believes that the early prevention and diagnosis of disease is the best way to enhance population health. The World Health Organization also believes that in the 21st century, "Disease-focused Medicine" will turn into "Health-focused Medicine", and will focus more on "Prevention" rather than "Treatment"[①]. "*Health China 2030 Plan*" has also pointed out that the core of Healthy China strategy is population health. Key statement includes "continuing focus on primary healthcare and prevention", "to promote wide participant, contribute to the construction of healthy China and move towards prevention-oriented healthcare", "Emphasis on early diagnosis, early treatment and early recovery, to achieve universal health". There are considerable investment benefits on early prevention and early diagnosis of disease. The study conducted by University of Columbia had confirmed that once the "early diagnosis" was strengthened, the national medical costs would be greatly reduced. For cardiovascular disease, for example, the United Kingdom, Germany and China can reduce 42% of the costs. The United States can also reduce 36%, about 142.4 billion USD. In the UK, most of the integrated healthcare models for the elderly are committed to integrating clinical and other medical services through population management tools. These population-based models capture information of the population and divide them into different risk groups through reliable and standardized

---

① Wang H C, Ma Z L, Lu C J. Research on the transformation of medical care mode[J]. Zizhi Wenzhai, 2009(1): 62—63.

approaches to achieve early detection. In the meanwhile, the UK has established different risk prediction models. They are used by institutions of the National Health Service (NHS). In addition to achieving early detection of cases, these tools can also be used for resource allocation among people, as well as performance management and evaluation. From a long-term perspective, it would be very helpful to establish a system of health education, prevention and management, through close communications between physicians and patients, better prevention screening, more effective management of high-risk patients and fine management of high healthcare expenses.

4.3　Use comprehensive interventions to avoid, or delay the admission and achieve early discharge

It is suggested to relay on institutional cooperation, adopting appropriate mechanisms, and encouraging conservation-oriented service patterns to reduce unreasonable hospitalization services for the elderly, avoid or delay admission, and encourage old persons to receive services in appropriate periods and content. The UK's experience of community based admissions avoidance and early supported discharge services could be usefully adapted to other systems of healthcare[①].

The existing health care system does not serve the elderly patient well. In the lack of a reasonable and orderly health-seeking order, many health problems that lead people to hospitalization are actually well resolved in the community, thus avoiding hospitalization. In fact, Western countries are building more service models that are based on community to provide service against acute symptoms. Taking Australia as an example, there are Hospital in the Home (HIH) and Hospital in the Nursing Home (HINH)[②], which provides medical and nursing service at home so that the patients do no need to stay in hospital. Findings have shown that HIH and HINH are safe, acceptable and efficient for specific patients and symptoms as an

---

① Pramod Prabhakaran, SHDRC Report: UK integrated care perspective (Draft), 2017.

② CRILLY J., CHABOYER W. & WALLIS M. A structure and process evaluation of an Australian hospital admission avoidance programme for aged care facility residents [J]. Journal of Advanced Nursing, 2012,68(2), 322—334.

alternative to acute hospitalization. In order to achieve this model, we must build effective referral mechanisms and communication strategies between agencies. As the aging of the population becomes increasingly severe, reducing admission rate of the elderly patient will have a significant impact on their health outcomes. It also reduces hospital-acquired complications, and allows the elderly to receive medical services in a favored environment.

4.4　Use nursing and rehabilitation as an alternative to acute treatment

It was found that in China, elderly nursing homes are facing great challenge on "bed occupation". A large number of elderly people who only need low-density medical care choose to stay in medical institutions. What's more, some elderly people are taking long-term nursing service in hospital and use existing medical insurance to pay for it. There are also reports showed that due to existing medical insurance, old people consider "district hospital is less expensive than nursing homes" thus they prefer to take a ward bed in hospital for pension purpose[1]. In fact, it is a huge threat to the medical insurance system to adopt elders with no therapeutic value in hospital. The elderly covered by Medical insurance often bring the cost of nursing services into medical insurance and medical assistance schemes in the name of the needs of medical care. Although it is legal for medical insurance fund to pay these expenses, it is not cost-effective at all[2]. The irrational transfer of these services squeezed the medical resources which are already limited and expensive, thus caused difficulties in access to medical services. International experience has shown that nursing and rehabilitation services can play a great role to replace hospital services. It also brings long-term benefits to elderly people's mental health. It is suggested to promote palliative care (hospice care) project and set up institutions and home soothing beds for the elderly in their end of life to provide hospice care. However, although the framework system already exists, the integration of resources is still to be developed, and the utilization of nursing and rehabilitation services is yet to be improved,

---

[1]　Xu Y J, Yang Y H, Yang G, et al. Questions and current situation of the elders' nursing care beds allocation in Shanghai[J]. Chinese Health Resources, 2014(3): 157—159.

[2]　Yang T. The policy choice of long-term care in China.

which calls the department concerned to integrate medical services resources and optimize the service structure for old people.

5. Improve equity and narrow down the differences between schemes

Social and economic environment directly or indirectly have influence on the elderly people's health. Environment's impact on the elderly people's health varies greatly because of individual difference (such as family background and gender). This leads to the inequality and inequity of health, especially to the elderly[1]. There are wide differences in capability and status quo of a number of elderly people, which is likely the cumulative advantage /disadvantage caused by all the health inequity in the life course[2]. Some studies revealed that the utilization of medical services is closely related to economic level, health status and level of medical insurance, etc. The diversity of related factors leads to the inequity of utilization of medical services and medical burden, which further have impact on the health inequity of elderly people[3][4]. The utilization of medical services and the costs of those services also show that the level of financing and reimbursement in the three systems of basic medical insurance vary considerably. Hence, it's necessary to promote the health equity of the elderly by financing, full use of service and many other ways.

5.1　Guarantee the health rights of the elderly

The improvement and perfection of health equity of the elderly should be carried forward together with serious and catastrophic disease insurance. Firstly, on the basis of fully implementing the Urban Residents Serious

---

① Commission on Social Determinants of Health. Closing the gap in a generation: health equity through action on social determinants of health. Final report of the Commission on Social Determinants of Health. Geneva: World Health Organization, 2008.

② Dannefer D. Cumulative advantage /disadvantage and the life course: cross-fertilizing age and social science theory. J Gerontol B Psychol Sci Soc Sci. 2003 Nov; 58 (6): S327-37.doi: ttp: //dx.doi.org/10.1093/geronb/58.6.S327 PMID: 14614120.

③ Chen P R, Wu L, Zhu L S, ect. Analysis of the utilization of health care and their influencing factors among the elderly: Based on CHARLS data[J]. Chinese Journal of Social Medicine,2015,32(2): 153—155.

④ Jie E. Research on inequality in health and medical services using revenue -related [J].Economic Research Journal,2009(2): 92—105.

Disease Insurance, the accuracy of paying for patients with serious disease who cannot afford medical cost should be increased by lowering the deductible, increasing the level of reimbursement and setting up a rational and compliant range of medical cost. Secondly, comprehensive medical help should be offered to people living on minimum subsistence allowance and extremely poor people. On this basis, the elderly people in low income family and patients with serious disease whose family suffers illness-caused poverty should also be involved in the list of being aided, which plays a vital role that aims to guarantee the right of those who live in poverty. Thirdly, several parties such as social charity forces are encouraged to make some contribution. A data-sharing mechanism between medical facilities and medical insurance agencies also should be established. Basic Medical Insurance, Serious Disease Insurance, Medical Assistance, Emergency Aid Commercial Health Insurance should be connected to each other closely and effectively to offer one-stop service in an all-round way.

5.2　Make comprehensive arrangements on the system of basic medical insurance and promote equity

Shanghai begins to implement Regulation on Urban and Rural Residents Basic Medical Insurance since 2016. It sets unified standard on coverage, financing policy, insurance incentives, medicine directory, management of designated medical institutions and fund. However, the disparity between the Urban Employee Basic Medical Insurance and the Urban and Rural Residents Basic Medical Insurance remains. They differ in financing and insurance incentives. It's suggested to make further comprehensive arrangements on Basic Medical Insurance and give priority to the equity of the elderly people's healthcare service in all systems and then ensure the equity of all. Firstly, stable and sustainable financing system should be established. The respective paying obligation of government, unit and individual should be clearly defined in the policy of medical insurance. When fiscal input is increased and favors the elderly, the subsidy standard is promoted. Meanwhile, the consciousness of individual insuring should be strengthened. If one who has the Urban Employee Basic Medical Insurance still has his/her account balance in black, he/she can subsidize his/her family member (especially the elderly) by the surplus to take out the Urban and Rural Residents Basic Medical Insurance. The different proportion of premiums the insurer needs to pay in different systems should be balanced. Secondly, a dynamic insurance incentive adjustment mechanism should be promoted and perfected, which is well adapted to the level of financing. Necessary steps include: (1) Make a clear and comprehensive definition on the range of basic medical insurance and standardize the incentive; (2) Encourage the sharing of individual insurance account within family; (3) Healthcare costs meeting relevant provisions can now be settled on the spot when incurred anywhere within the provincial-level administrative area where insurance is registered. Under such circumstance, promote and lay emphasis on distributing more medical resources to basic levels and propel the establishment of medical treatment combination. Set up a hierarchical treatment regime and ensure rational convergence and coordination within different levels. Thirdly, medical insurance handling capacity should be developed. More innovative measures should be taken in medicine purchasing, cost clearing, negotiation on medical insurance payment standard and agreement management and account settlement of designated medical institutions. Medical insurance should play a role in controlling the unreasonable growth of medical costs to promote system equity.

5.3　Build a theoretical framework of health equity based on the outcome

The universal medical insurance system can help to change old ideas that the former basic medical insurance system relied on, such as the principle of choosing and identity discrimination. It can also prevent from the cost transfer among personnel in different systems and embody modern values of welfare, including popularized and whole-of-population approach, equality, civil rights, basic needs and health priority[1]. With the advancement of universal medical insurance, health equity means the equity of right and need that lies both in the process and in the result instead of opportunity equity, whether one has the insurance or not. It's a unity of individual rights and responsibilities that the government must undertake.

---

① Liu J T. "One system, diversified standards" and the whole people's fundamental medical treatment insurance system frame[J]. Journal Of Humanities, 2006, (3): 7—13.

Equity consists of horizontal equity and vertical equity. Horizontal equity in medical care insurance is divided into 3 dimensions: equity in range (coverage), equity in width (insurance content) and equity in height (insurance incentive). It requires the equal treatment of people in the same situation. On the other hand, vertical equity requires various levels of insurance in accordance with different medical service demands. But all these measures can only guarantee the equity in the process. An equitable health outcome is more important. To build a theoretical framework of health equity based on the outcome, the target of policy should be clearly set. The target should be shifted from input to output and — better yet — outcome[1], including improved health status, quality of care, patients' satisfaction, and reduction of patients' economic burden. Secondly, based on the elderly people's healthcare needs, medical costs and care costs should both be compensated. The overall health equity of the elderly during the whole process can be promoted by connecting and integrating prevention, treatment, rehabilitation, nursing care and end-of-life care together on the principle of "same need, same treatment". Thirdly, to promote the process equity, the input in basic medical treatment and public health should be increased and the allocation of medical resources can be perfected by transfer payment, adoption of preferential policy and other measures. All these actions aim to achieve the equitable outcome of the elderly people's health.

6. Formulate targeted burden-relieving policy and provide financial protection

6.1 Protect the patients with a serious disease from over-heavy burden

According to a ranking of hospitalization costs for diseases among the elderly in Shanghai in 2015, the top three diseases were cardiovascular diseases, malignances and respiratory diseases with higher gross hospitalization cost and patient co-payment per visit. Therefore, the Urban Employee Basic Medical Insurance has established a system to alleviate the

---

① Yip W C, Hsiao W C, Chen W, et al. Early appraisal of China's huge and complex health-care reforms[J]. Lancet, 2012, 379(9818): 833—842.

overall burden on patients and meanwhile the Urban Residents Basic Medical Insurance features serious disease insurance to reduce the medical expenses borne by patients with a serious disease. The cost burden of all the patients who have the serious disease insurance is effectively alleviated. The proportion of compensation for four types of diseases (dialysis for severe uremia, anti-rejection therapy after a kidney transplant, treatment of malignancies, and treatment of some psychiatric illnesses) rises by 23 percent ~ 24 percent on average. The diseases covered are limited. For instance, chronic diseases such as stroke which makes the elderly overburdened and rare diseases that bring serious burden are all not covered. The reimbursement cost of serious disease insurance accounts for 0.5% of the whole expenditure of the Urban Resident Medical Insurance in 2015. Balance of the Urban Resident Medical Insurance had amounted to 410 million Yuan by 2016 (17.1% of that year's fund revenue) while the reimbursement cost of serious disease insurance accounts for 3.2% of the cumulative fund revenue. There is still a large amount of fund precipitation. To further improve the availability of serious disease insurance, the following action can be taken:

Firstly, the scope of covered serious diseases in Shanghai should be gradually expanded based on the data from epidemiology and burden of disease. The Serious Disease Insurance scheme now covers 4 types of disease. But the scope of covered disease can be expanded in accordance with prevalence, the length of the course of the disease, and its costs. The targeted policy should be formulated to alleviate the overall burden on the elderly patients with serious disease who cannot bear the treatment cost. Serious disease insurance covers dialysis for severe uremia, anti-rejection therapy after a kidney transplant, treatment of malignancies, and treatment of some psychiatric illnesses. The diseases covered are limited. As an example, cardiovascular disease is most prevalent among the elderly and incurs the largest hospitalization costs but is not covered. In principle, the scope of covered diseases needs to be expanded in accordance with prevalence, the length of the course of the disease, and its costs.

Secondly, costs should be the main factor in determination of serious illness. If a serious disease is defined in accordance to its type, it results in easier operation and the control over costs also becomes easier, beneficial to the safe running of the fund. However, many of the patients who bear high medical expenses have diseases that are not involved in the policy. When the medical cost is rather high or even exceeds the high medical cost standard that set by the policy in a certain period of time, the disease can be regarded as serious disease. Defining serious disease based on the cost can reduce the possibility of falling into poverty or being reduced to poverty due to illness and is more equitable. Since the present policy that relies on types of diseases for definition could give patients with great medical cost burden a leg-up, defining serious illness bases on the cost could serve as a supplementary method. Hence, the cost standard should be properly improved. The coverage of insurance can be expanded and the standard can be reduced until financing fund is enough.

Thirdly, set up patient co-payment maximum line. Maximum payment instead of patient co-payment maximum line is set in our country's medical insurance payment system. This aims to protect from the risk of balance-of-payments other than the risk of patients' disease. Then it results in a situation that low-income groups and those who suffer serious diseases still cannot afford the medical treatment. Public health resources they should enjoy are taken advantage of by other groups. It is advised to set up the patient co-payment maximum line and income level (the equity that must be achieved) according to the economic development level. The pooling fund will pay surplus medical expenses that exceed the patient co-payment maximum line. People with catastrophic disease or particular difficulty will be offered further medical insurance assistance or reduction and exemption of cost.

6.2　Reduce non-direct medical costs through long-term care insurance and subsidy

The sample data conducted by China Health and Retirement Longitudinal Study shows the proportion of aging population with a loss of capacity in different age group in China. 16.37% of the elderly people aged 60 and over have lost their living capability in 2011. With the fast growth of aging population in China, it is estimated that the amount of the elderly with a loss of capacity will have reached 57.44 million by 2030 and the cost produced by the great need for elderly care will have reached 2.1 trillion

Yuan, 1.7% of 2030's GDP. However, the great need for elderly care cannot be transformed into the utilization of elderly care in reality because the average low income and the low consumption rate of the elderly make the transformation less feasible at present. Historical data shows that the elderly in China mainly depend on their family member, earned income and pensions. Even the elderly living in a city with higher level of insurance cannot pay for the elderly care whose cost is getting higher and higher because their pensions can only cover 76% of their daily costs. Meanwhile, scarcely can the cost of care service to the elderly people with a loss of capability be reimbursed, directly leading to a high non-medical cost. The research has once interviewed an acute cerebral infarction patient with a prolonged stay in hospital. His daily cost for employing a care worker for the whole day reached 210 Yuan. This implicit cost is not shown in the medical cost bill and the patient's family has to cover it on their own. It will lead to a heavy economic burden on patients' family in the long run. In addition, long-term care service will also bring great pressure to a family. The elderly in our country mainly depend on home nursing. Some of the old people have difficulty in standing or cannot stand for a long period of time because of their old age or chronic disease. They also lose the basic self-care ability in daily life and have to rely on care-giver, which brings great pressure to family care. What's more, care givers are faced with great challenge as some of them are also in bad health and some of them have to work as well as raise their young.

Long-term care insurance that offers reimbursement of care service cost should be established as soon as possible. A perfect community health care system and a comprehensive supporting system that combine hospital, community and family together should be established. These systems aim to help the elderly people with a loss of capability and care-givers fully achieve the community medical treatment, health service resources, instruct other family members to share the care work together with the care-giver and give the care-giver support psychologically, materially and physically. They also help the care-giver emphasize on the relation between his/her own health and care work, offering more emotional and mental support. Furthermore, care reimbursement should also be offered to family caregivers through insurance or public finance to encourage home nursing and alleviate economic burden of family care-givers.

7. Promote social service and emphasize humanistic care

The management of medical care and community care in UK belongs respectively to two different government departments, the Ministry of Health and local authority. There used to be the problem of incoherent service. Shanghai as well as the whole nation meets with the same challenge: medical health and aging service are managed by the department of health and department of civil administration. Services and payment work incoherently. In December, 2013, the State Council issued the Several Opinions on Accelerating the Development of Elderly Care Service Industry (No. 35 in 2013). The Opinions originally put forward the notion of the co-development of medical service and care service. After that, Shanghai government also point out that "propel the establishment of social elderly care service" to meet the diversified needs of the elderly in Implementation Opinions of Accelerating the Development of Elderly Care Service Industry and the Construction of Social Elderly Service issued in April, 2014 (No. 28 in 2014).

7.1 Make comprehensive arrangements on social service and promote the development of nursing care system

In 2002, NHS in Britain introduced Integrated Care Trusts to offer better integrated medical health services and social services. Now some regions are launching a pilot project that combines the budgets of health service and social service while at the same time integrates the management framework and manages health and social service in community together. Following suggestion is made for developing social service. (1) Daily Life. The social services provided to the elderly should meet their needs in life and help to eliminate dangerous factors, alleviate disease burden, and lower the possibility of emergency and hospitalization. Then it can also help save resources and increase the level of health. In addition, efforts should be actively made to get the support of the department of finance for the services that are greatly needed by some of the elderly. Then these services can be offered to citizens in form of practical projects of the municipal government. For example, Japan has involved social service projects like the lease of assistive devices and transformation of houses to be barrier-free in its long-term care insurance. Similar pilot project can be launched step by step and region by region. The lease of assistive devices for the elderly people with a loss of capability can be run in a way as that of the public bicycles leasing that is quite popular in various cities. (2) Community. The service resources within the region can be reasonably allocated in accordance with demand assessment of the elderly care which is promoted in the 16 districts in Shanghai. One or several managers of the integrated service system can be appointed on the level of community to be responsible for management of medical health and social service in the whole community. (3) Society. The government should lead the development of social services and families and the whole society should also participate in the development. The collaboration among government, social organizations and other social forces are advocated in principle. Their cooperation and co-management can help to maximize the public benefit. By encouraging social organizations to offer social service, the dispersed service resources can be effectively combined together and the service efficiency can be improved. (4) Development direction. Some regions in Britain have already completed the budget integration of health and social service. But in Shanghai, the barriers between different government departments are quite difficult to break through. A list of the most needed services by the elderly can be made with the help of long-term care insurance which is now piloted. The social service can be supported through payment. To develop social service not only needs the efforts made by the department of civil administration, but also needs to learn from Britain's experience, strengthen the interactive mechanism among the departments of health, civil administration and medical insurance. Therefore, the social service can be integrated into the whole social elderly care service system.

7.2　Strengthen the social support and explore an appropriate end-of-life care model

In 2004, Britain unveiled its "End of Life Care Plan" and made End of Life Care Strategy across Britain in 2008. The government focused on building the end of life care system under top-level design, launched in-depth investigation into end-of-life for several times and put forward

"Ambitions for Palliative and End of Life Care: A national framework for local action 2015—2020". Setting up palliative care (end of life care) bed is one of the ways that Shanghai carries out its end of life work. The work was deeply implemented in 2012 and 2014 as a practical project of the municipal government. There are more than 1,700 palliative care beds in 76 medical agencies (mainly the community healthcare center) that provide palliative treatment and care service for old people and dying patients in need. According to the experience of Britain, end of life care system helps to save medical costs and promote health performance. There are two main points that is important in building a more appropriate end of life care model. Firstly, an end of life care model that makes family, community and medical staff work together should be established. This model should recognize who are the elderly people in last stage and patients in end stage in need for end of life care. People himself and his family members also have the right to know and to decide. If one chooses to spend his last phase of life on the basic palliative care bed, his family, the community and medical staff should coordinate with each other and take their own responsibilities. Secondly, equal emphasis should be laid on the elderly people's physical and psychological health. On the one hand, end of life care relieves the pain of body by medical technology and help the patient die peacefully. On the other hand, spiritual concern and spirit guide are also important. For those who have religion, religion can help to overcome their fear and let them face death in a right manner.

The disease treatment and alleviation of pain are as important as psychological counseling and humanistic care. The social service should be organically combined with health care, working together to ensure the elderly to enjoy in old age well. End of life care is an indispensable part in the whole medical health system. The end of life care system should be constructed at the city level and an overall objective should be established to lay the foundation for perfection of medical healthcare system, saving of medical resources and increase of system running efficiency.

8. Develop a management tool for the elderly with the use of big data

That mass unstructured data is a challenge that faced by the elderly medical care industry. The analysis of big data helps to improve the medical efficiency, create additional value and then achieve better outcomes. In 2015, the State Council issued an action outline to promote the development of big data. This outline put it forward that the goal of promoting the opening, sharing, convergence and integration of medical big data is to solve the problem of Data Island and service isolation that exists in the current elderly medical care industry. Active steps can be taken to tackle aging, such as eliminating information technology obstacles and data sharing obstacles, integrating the agency-centered system framework and developing diversified elderly-oriented data management tools and applying the result of data analysis.

8.1　Promote data sharing within different organizations and optimize the data collection

The establishment of Shanghai health big data platform mainly depends on Shanghai Municipal Commission of Health and Family Planning Information Center. It launches a project of health information network which focuses on the health management of citizens. Now it forms a data center that connects the information of "1 + 18" regions (city center, medical union and 17 district centers).

In order to make the exchange and sharing of elderly care information possible, the first thing to do is to break up the limitation on interactivity across systems and break down the barriers within different organizations. Barriers include the following factors. (1) Horizontal barriers among government departments. The fragmentation that data respectively collected by the department of police, health, social insurance, civil administration and disabled should be changed. (2) Vertical barriers among government departments. The municipal and regional platforms should be linked and data should be transferred at fixed time. Before that, a unified standard or regulation of information collection should be set. Data integration department should also use the same data transmission tool to make sure that the information of the elderly collected from different channels can be uniquely identified and reused. More efforts should be made to improve the quality of data. Taking Britain as an example, Spine is the database of NHS patients' information which stores the name, gender, age, home address and other basic information of patients as well as medical records. Further information such as use of medication, allergic history and adverse drug reaction is also recorded in the extended national record center. Information can be transmitted to anywhere u emergency through network. The medical staff can look over the records when authorized. The information can be safely shared by Electronic Prescription Service, Summary Care Records, and e-Referral Service①. Furthermore, it's worth noting that information collection is only developed in public medical institutions. Private institutions like nursing homes are not involved, not to mention the informal care offered by family members. When home nursing is advocated, the data in this field is an important part that needs to be taken into consideration in later reform.

8.2　Develop diversified risk stratification tools and promote the assessment of long-term care needs of the elderly

Most medical institutions prefer to invest in the promotion of interior management efficiency but rarely consider involving patients' information in their information system. Apply the results of big data analysis to the elderly medical care service is much more rare. With the help of advanced information technology and mass big data, a management tool that based on population can be developed. This helps to improve the efficiency of using existed information, making the elderly medical care more accurate and more personalized. When the society is devoted to offer integrated medical care services, a set of reliable and standardized Risk Stratification Tools can be developed with the information from hospitals and community health centers. Based on the Risk Score that updates dynamically, the medical staff can determine the groups of high risks in a certain period of time, predict the group whose Risk Score is ascending. Besides, these management tools can effectively support the reasonable distribution of medical care resources in different aging groups and promote performance management and assessment. For example, Britain has established a Dementia Data Extract project targeting Alzheimer, which aims to collect the information of elderly people from general practice, so that they can

---

① NHS Digital. Spine. https://digital.nhs.uk/spine.

find out the group at the risk of having Alzheimer. Meanwhile, the project also extracts the information of Alzheimer patients' visit to hospital and services they receive. With the unified assessment tool, general practitioners can conduct professional evaluation of the elderly and keep tracking the information timely to ensure an early detection and intervention[1]. One case of Shanghai data management tool is the needs assessment of the elderly care. This assessment covers the aging group and collects information on respondents themselves and their family, activities of daily living, mental health, emotion, mental health and disease diagnosis. It's expected to grade them into different levels in accordance with the assessment results and then provide different care service for the elderly.

8.3　Accelerate the analysis and application of big data with the use of information technology

Health is a comprehensive and successive concept. The health condition in older stage is largely connected to the history of disease at every life stage. Hence, the elderly medical care service is retrospective. When data sharing and management is strengthened at early phase, a more comprehensive and updated electronic health records can be established, helping the medical staff get command of health information of the elderly at all stages. An upgraded analysis on the electronic health records can help to further identify the elderly who are the susceptible population of a certain disease. The medical staff can better supervise the care services and offer predictive service by the analysis. The electronic records are also helpful in finding the most suitable care plan from existing health management plans. The records should be moveable and editable, easy for patients and their caregivers to reach. In addition, with the development of information technology, the application of big data can be accelerated and the elderly patients with chronic disease can get remote health supervision service with high-tech outfits and wearable devices. They can consult general practitioners via video, get prescription and look for the complete

---

① NHS Digital. Dementia data extract. https: //digital. nhs. uk /GP-Collections / service-information /dementia-data-extract.

electronic health records online. Therefore, the medical resources can be freed and the elderly can supervise their health by themselves. The health resource investment, to some extent, can be saved also.

To sum up, the hidden value of big data should be discovered in order to cope with aging effectively. Data should be integrated so that it can be shared and compared. With the help of data, information and technology, the healthy and sustainable development of elderly care service can be promoted by the following means: design a modern management model that based on populations and develop valuable Risk Stratification Tools; make scientific assessment on health conditions of the elderly and grade them into different levels in accordance with the assessment results; provide diversified medical care service and make reasonable distribution of resources and introduce social security policies.

9. Implement specific strategies to deal with the priority disease and injuries

Specific strategy aiming at the diseases with high morbidity rate among the elderly people and significant physical and psychological impact to the elderly should be established.

9.1 The strategy of dementia

According to the 2015 World Alzheimer Report[1], there are 46 million people worldwide suffering from Alzheimer's disease. This number is greater than the entire population of the country of Spain, and the number of patients with dementia will be more than 130 million by 2050. In China, in 2010, the proportion of $65 \sim 69$ year-old elderly people suffering from senile dementia is 2.6%, and the proportion of $95 \sim 99$ years old group reached 60.5%[2]. Analysis showed that, the study of disease burden based on small sample in the past might have underestimated the burden of

---

①　Alzheimer's Disease International, World Alzheimer Report 2015 – The Global Impact of Dementia: An analysis of prevalence, incidence, cost and trends, https: // www.alz.co.uk/research/WorldAlzheimerReport2015.pdf

②　Chan KY, Wang W, Wu JJ, et al. Epidemiology of Alzheimer's disease and other forms of dementiain China, 1990—2010: a systematic review and analysis [J]. Lancet, 2013, 381(9882): 2016—2023.

dementia in China, and dementia disease burden growth rate is faster than the expected rate by international community. The government needs to take prompt and effective responses to the problem of dementia in low and middle income countries. Firstly, it should enhance public awareness of dementia, and establish a dignified, independent and inclusive social support system. Secondly, it should improve availability of service, establish a "Task Sharing" service model, put the majority of care service into the process of primary care and community service, non-professionals trained by professionals and supported by them while carry out the service. Thirdly, it should control risk factors. Regarding the risk factors analysis for dementia, the most likely risk factors are the low level of early education, suffering from high blood pressure in middle age, as well as the smoking behavior during entire life process and diabetes history[1]. More studies have shown that the risk of dementia can be reduced. Further research and health promotion actions are needed[2][3]. The first step to implement dementia risk factors control is to let more people know, dementia can be prevented to some extent. Finally, it should pay attention to patients' family services, as this could have a positive impact on people's health and reduce the costs of society. Meanwhile, medical assistive skills and home care services should be further developed to delay the patients admitted to hospital.

9.2　The specific strategy to prevent falls

Fall is the leading causes of disability, the primary cause of death among the elderly people about 75-year-olds, and is the top priority issue for the elderly

---

① Prince M, Albanese E, Guerchet M, et al. World Alzheimer Report 2014. Dementia and Risk Reduction. An analysis of Protective and Modifiable Risk Factors. London: Alzheimer's Disease International, 2014.

② Lincoln P, Fenton K, Alessi C, et al. The Blackfriars Consensus on brain health and dementia [J]. Lancet, 2014, 383(9931): 1805—1806.

③ Norton S, Matthews F E, Barnes D E, et al. Potential for primary prevention of Alzheimer's disease: An analysis of population-based data [J]. Lancet, 2014, 13(8): 788—794.

health, and is regulated in many nations' service framework①. Each year, about 420,000 people die from falls, of which over 80% occur in low and middle income countries. The ability to prevent falls and support elderly people to regain their independent lives has been a challenge for many health and social service organizations. The strategy to prevent falls should emphasize health education, training, and create a safer environment, prioritize research related to falls, and formulate effective policies to reduce risk.

Column 1 Britain falls prevention services started since 2004, Oxfordshire provided this service by integrating Radcliffe hospital emergency services and the services provided by community health and volunteer organizations, reducing the incidence rate of old people falling in this county, improving the life quality of the elderly who fall and the people at high risk. This model integrates the professional skills of a number of different disciplines to form a multi-disciplinary service team, including: emergency services, physiotherapists, occupational therapists, fall related professional nurses, motor coordination professionals. Provided services including: training for staff in the nursing home and evaluation of fall injury; to improve people's understanding and attention of the fall in the related fields of all the health and social services; posting information about fall injury medical institutions and service team; providing related consulting and exercise program for the elderly in community and hospital; providing the balance and security project in the daytime service agencies; providing preventive measures project for the high-risk population; providing uninterrupted technical support and advice for related services personnel under the support of acute care hospitals professional team; cooperating with emergency services, to improve

---

① Department of Health. National service framework for older people[EB/OL]. (2015-12-21). http://www.gov.uk/government/uploads/system/uploads/attachment_data/file/19803 3/National_Service_Framework_for_Older_People.pdf.

the quality of health care services for the fall by providing ways such as referral, fall prevention and reduction of ambulance service call frequency. This referral services can be derived from several aspects, including service users and their families or caregivers. Provide people-centered and personalized service response for the special needs of the individual. It can refer the elderly to a physical exercise project, occupational therapy, psychological treatment, and hospital treatment or general practitioner service project according to the specific situation.

9.3　The strategy of Parkinson's disease

China is in a sharp rise stage of the number of patients with Parkinson's disease, excluding changes in the morbidity of Parkinson's disease, the population aging is the most important reason. Results of a study in 2007 showed that in the current and future period of time, the number of patients with Parkinson's disease in China will account for about half of the world: In 2005, the number of cases of Parkinson's disease in China is about 1.99×10^6 cases, the worldwide number is about 4.10×10^6 cases; in 2030 the number of cases of Parkinson's disease in China will be about 4.94×10^6 cases, the worldwide number is about 8.67×10^6[①]. Firstly, it should establish evidence-based treatment guidelines for Parkinson's disease. Through the development and dissemination of guidelines, health technology assessment and decision-making transformation as well as relevant training and promotion work, the government should help professionals adopt more standardized and appropriate health technologies, so as to provide residents with better health services. Secondly, it should employ professionals to build up local area network of professional services, review and adapt high professional standards and highly motivated professionals of healthcare and health insurance, to enable patients consult with their long-term treatment recommendation. The professionals involved

---

① Liu S Y, Chen B. Epidemiology of Parkinson's disease[J]. Chinese Journal of Contemporary Neurology and Neurosurgery, 2016 (2): 98—101.

include neurologist, home care specialists, rehabilitation specialists, psychiatrists, psychologists, pharmacists, nurses specialized in Parkinson's disease, behavioral therapist, the conversation-speech therapists, dietitians and social workers. Thirdly, it should introduce Internet technology to establish health service platform. The government should take advantage of Internet technology to face the current medical challenge, build knowledge platform for chronic disease management based on the whole management process, help patients with chronic diseases and high-risk groups to achieve self-management through this platform, increase the percentage of their awareness and control of chronic diseases, and realize precise health promotion.

9.4 The strategy of stroke

Stroke is an acute cerebrovascular disease with high morbidity rates in the elderly population, due to the high incidence rate, high mortality rate, high disability rate, and it has attracted the attention from the health care sector and the whole society. It is suggested that the clinical characteristics of stroke should be combined with multiple disciplines and sectors to establish prevention and treatment network. And it should be fully combined with the characteristics of the elderly people, targeted to establish the elderly green channel for stroke treatment. First of all, it should be combined with civil affairs departments, and vigorously strengthen stroke prevention and control knowledge among the elderly people, advocate healthy lifestyle, control stroke risk factors, to strengthen the identification of stroke symptoms. For high-risk groups, such as hypertension, diabetes mellitus elderly patients should establish special program to carry out the propaganda of stroke knowledge and the promotion of awareness of health management. Secondly, in the hospital, it should explore to establish green channel for patients with acute cardiovascular and cerebrovascular diseases, strengthen the cohesion between the emergency department and clinical departments. At present, because of the restrictions of the medical treatment system, it lacks coordination among departments in the course of stroke diagnosis and treatment, timely treatment need to be enhanced. It is recommended to break the single-disciplinary stroke treatment model, to provide the elderly patients individualized, standardized and comprehensive treatment and intervention. At the same time, it is recommended to establish a closed-loop for stroke rescue and treatment which is started from community to the hospital and then back to the community, to provide integrated services including screening of high-risk population and medical, rehabilitation, care, psychological and other needs in different aspects for stroke patients. Regarding the characteristics of the elderly people, we suggest to plan and design transport and traffic roadway for stroke patients, which can further improve the timeliness of rescue and the convenience of rehabilitation.

Column 2 It has become a trend in the development of medical industry that promotes the effective practice of prevention and control of chronic diseases by assisting chronic disease management personnel in managing patients with chronic disease.UK Parkinson's Excellence Network integrates medical resources at all levels to build "online service platform" leaded by large public hospital medical service, and based on the primary care and community health service. It makes health resources of all levels interact with each other and provides quality health services for Parkinson's patients practically and effectively. Dutch Parkinson Net established a specialized information technology platform, it includes: a specialized web with search engine, as well as a network BBS for patients and professionals, they can communicate with each other directly on the platform. Aiming at patients, Parkinson Net provides a decision support tool, and the patient can find important background information through this link, such as: the effects and evidences of different treatment strategies in Parkinson's disease, so as to make the patients to participate in decision-making. Patients can also consult via video link in their own homes. One of the Parkinson Net's key objectives is to improve the transparency of the treatment quality that the patients received, therefore it needs to open the data of the quality of treatment to the public. For example: Parkinson Atlas (Atlas www. Parkinson. Nl) shows relevant information from the perspective of Parkinson.net in different areas, such as medical costs, admission rate of hospital or rehabilitation center, the quality of the cooperation among disciplines. The patients BBS can help promote the quality of the follow-up treatment. For example, patients use "wiki" (an application website that allows users to work with others to add, edit or delete content) to create useful information entry in living with Parkinson's disease, and discuss the quality evaluation of the treatment that patients received and auxiliary treatment experience. Aiming at the medical professionals, Parkinson Net provides an online BBS, it makes the experts in the BBS communicate with each other conveniently, facilitate them to exchange experiences with each other and communicate with each other in terms of new information of treatment technology.

10. Strengthen relevant measures and form forceful government support

With the deepening of aging population degree in China, aging will become a new social ecology. The health condition and functional ability of the elderly depend on the medical service system as well as natural and social environment. Several fields and various social roles are involved in the process of building an environment of healthy aging. Government at all levels and every department concerned need to take actions together. *Healthy China 2030* put forward that health should be combined into all major policies. Five major tasks include promoting healthy lifestyles, optimizing health services, perfecting health care system, developing health industry and building a healthy environment. All the departments and fields should cooperate with each other to promote health under the guidance of these five tasks.

10.1 Reinforce the collaboration in all fields from four different aspects

Leading Group Office of Social Elderly Care Service Construction was set up in Shanghai, which aims to coordinate the development of aging industry, and lead the cooperation within different departments and regions to deal with aging. The work includes setting goals and tasks, clarifying responsibilities, securing budget and establishing a mechanism that ensures the cooperation, monitoring, assessment and reporting within departments. The collaboration can be achieved in four aspects. (1) The horizontal collaboration among government departments. This involves different agencies and departments belong to the same level of government collaborating across missions and jurisdictions. For instance, the planning and construction of elderly medical institutions and nursing homes require the cooperation between the department of city planning and health. The construction of related facilities for the elderly (for example, construct accessible toilets or build walking paths) also needs the collaboration among civil administration department, road administration department, quality supervision department and committee of aging population. (2) The vertical collaboration among government departments. Municipal government and district government share the same goal and task and collaborate with each other. The district government implements the unified planning made by the municipal government and makes sure that the implementation is effective. (3) The cooperation between government departments and private sectors. Private sectors include non-governmental organizations, private industry and academic institutions. Government departments can cooperate with academic institution in launching the health intervention of the elderly. Public health institution, together with private agencies can work on medical treatment and nursing care for the elderly. (4) Cooperation between the government and families. The government can provide the informal caregiver with free training in order to enhance the elderly people's quality of life and functional abilities.

10.2　Establish a health-need-oriented mechanism of investment and incentive

Firstly, an outcome-oriented health investment system should be established and the performance of health investment should be supervised and assessed. The WHO report divides the elderly into three stages according to functional abilities: high and stable, declining, and significant loss. The resource and fund investment should firstly be used to guarantee the public health service, preventing the elderly from having diseases or reduce the risk of diseases. An early detection and treatment of non-communicable diseases are also an area in which action can be taken. Secondly, the health investment at grass roots level should be increased. Effective disease management and health service should be offered to people with, or at high risk for, cardiovascular diseases, cancers, chronic respiratory diseases, diabetes or other non-communicable disease. It can prevent the accumulation of functional deficit, and reduce the need for hospitalization and costly high-technology interventions. Thirdly, a common goal should be set and the efficiency of fund gathering and using should be improved. The department of civil administration gives aids in accordance with income other than medical need while the department of health focuses on the disease and the need for medical service, but fails to give priority to the actual need of the elderly. The two departments tend to arrange financial funds based on their established priorities, ignoring the real need. Cost-effective technologies and methods should be given more emphasis. Short-term and long-term policy objectives should be synthesized and clarified. A unified assessment tool should be used to carry out health care needs assessment. Stratified services and accurate management should be offered to the elderly. Finally, limited health insurance funds should be used to achieve precise protection through the optimization of institutional arrangements. Minimize the disease burden of the frail elderly who are in the low economic status and have high demand for medical services. Through the improvement of major health insurance system and exploration of the ceiling of patient co-payment, reasonable demand for medical care services could be protected.

10.3 Strengthen the capacity building and the management of human resources

A key characteristic of elderly disease is the high incidence of co-morbidities. Among the population aged 60 and above in Shanghai, 51.3% have four or more than four kinds of diseases. This determines the need for diagnosis and treatment across disciplines for the elderly. The diagnosis and treatment of serious and rare disease is needed as well as basic services like long-term care and rehabilitation. The various demands which result from the individual difference of the elderly require the medical staff to be omnipotent. Preferential policies on authorized size, career development and salary should be made in order to attract and retain suitable talents. First, introduce and cultivate talents that can "hold up the heavens". Shanghai is establishing the Geriatrics Medical Center. The cultivation and introduction of high level talents can help to propel the construction of geriatrics, helping to reach the leading position within the country and in the world. Second, elderly service should "support the earth". The medical service of the elderly focuses on the need of collaboration between multiple disciplines and general practitioners. Education and training of the medical staff should no longer center on the treatment of acute diseases, but develop an integrated view that is elderly-oriented and emphasize on the management of chronic diseases. The cultivation of general practitioners should be reinforced and the ability to provide comprehensive service for the elderly should be improved. The personnel of nursing and rehabilitation which is in shortage should also be trained.

10.4 Promote the government collaboration and supervision through information construction

Institutional database should be well established, including basic information of elderly care institutions, medical care structure and cost. Similar to the display of parking spaces, publishing the distribution of elderly health care resources and the intensity of service utilization by GIS technology. This is beneficial for the patients to choose health institutions rationally and conveniently. Collaborated personal health database and health information platform that covers the whole population's whole life cycle should be well developed. The platform collects personal health information, assessment results of medical care demand, treatment and prescription information. All information should be interconnected. Data in different information systems including public health, medical service and insurance should be integrated and shared, promoting the connection between different service providers, enabling the elderly to have coherent treatment and improve the integrated efficiency and outcome. The government department can apply "information and technology" method to supervise the behavior of service providers and patients timely and dynamically. Prolonged hospitalization stays, frequent outpatient visits and high medical costs should be monitored. The rationality and value of medical services should be carefully assessed.

Older life stage is a normal but important phase of life. Respond to the aging society actively requires joint effort from society, industry and individual. With the help of information technology and the optimized system and the implementation of ten strategies, we can lessen or prevent injuries and regulate chronic diseases efficiently. Strengthen the elderly care service for disabled people, join forces to maintain and promote healthy aging and make the elderly better off.

Expand the financing channels and optimize financing mechanism. The source of medical insurance fund should be broadened and long-term insurance should be developed. An incentive and restriction mechanism should be established by setting paying levers and reforming on payment methods.

Change the medical service model into elderly-health-oriented. More attention should be paid on the intervention in residents' behavior and life style. A horizontally and vertically integrated medical service model should be built within the organization and the personalized medical service should be developed based on different needs.

Strengthen the resource distribution and put emphasis on the overall arrangement, integration and perfection. In the aspect of allocation, the resource distribution of elderly care based on big data should be implemented; With regard to the use of fund, we should co-ordination all resources through long-term care insurance; Concerning to the institutional resources, multiple kinds of integration and adjustments between medical institutions and nursing homes should be encouraged; Regarding to the personnel, we should strengthen the human resource development and training.

Promote the rational use of medical services and control medical expenses effectively. Irrational utilization of medical services should be mainly monitored and prolonged hospitalizations, frequent outpatient visits and high medical costs should also be monitored. Unnecessary medical treatments should be prevented by appropriate referral and redirection. The medical costs can be reduced by the change of medical service model.

Hospitalization can be avoided or delayed and the hospital discharge can be sooner by comprehensive intervention. Nursing and rehabilitation can act as a substitute on the treatment of acute diseases.

Improve equity and narrow down the differences between different systems. The health right of the elderly should be primarily protected. Basic medical insurance scheme should be fully arranged to improve equity. A theoretical framework of health equity based on the outcome should be built.

Formulate targeted burden-relieving policy and protect from financial risks. The scope of major disease insurance should be expanded and a ceiling of patient co-payment should be set up to prevent the patient from heavy burden due to catastrophic diseases. The indirect medical costs can be reduced by care insurance and financial subsidies.

Promote social service and emphasize humanistic care. Make comprehensive arrangements on social service and promote the development of elderly care service system. Social support should be strengthened and an appropriate end-of-life care model should be developed.

Develop a management tool for the elderly with the help of big data. Promote data sharing within different organizations and perfect the data collection. Accelerate the analysis and application of big data by information technology. Diversified Risk Stratification Tools can be developed to assist long-term care assessment.

Lead a special program to cope with key diseases and injuries. For the high morbidity of the elderly and its great influence on their functional and mental health, special programs such as Alzheimer Program, Parkinson Program, Stroke Program and falling prevention program should be launched.

Improve the supporting measures and make joint effort from governments. Co-ordinate the development of aging industry, lead the cooperation within different departments and regions to deal with aging. This work includes setting goals and tasks, clarifying responsibilities, securing budget and establishing a mechanism that ensures the cooperation, monitoring, assessment and reporting within departments.

参考文献

中文文献

[1] 陈春燕,罗羽,谢容.当前我国临终关怀模式存在的问题及对策[J].护理管理杂志,2005,5(2)：26—28.

[2] 陈雷.德国养老长期照护政策：目标、资金及给付服务内涵[J].中国民政,2016,(17)：36—37.

[3] 陈珉惺,王力男,杨燕,等.完善上海市基本医疗保险体系研究：基于商业健康保险视角[J].中国卫生政策研究,2015,8(11)：52—56.

[4] 陈培榕,吴拉,朱丽莎.老年人医疗服务利用及其影响因素分析——基于中国健康与养老追踪调查的数据[J].中国社会医学杂志,2015,32(2)：153—155.

[5] 陈翔,王小丽. 德国社会医疗保险筹资、支付机制及其启示[J].卫生经济研究,2009(12)：20—22.

[6] 崔娟,毛凡,王志会.中国老年居民多种慢性病共存状况分析[J].中国公共卫生,2016(1)：66—69.

[7] 丁汉升,杜丽侠,赵薇,等.上海市老年护理需求、费用及存在问题研究[J].老龄科学研究,2014(2)：47—53.

[8] 董国蕊,陈丽.医院药品费用占比的分析与调控[J].现代药物与临床,2012,27(6)：602—605.

[9] 方雨. 荷兰长期照护保险制度述评[J]. 中国医疗保险,2015（5）：68—70.

[10] 封进,余央央,楼平易.医疗需求与中国医疗费用增长——基于城乡老

年医疗支出差异的视角[J].中国社会科学,2015(3)：85—103.

[11]　郭斌.上海市居家养老医疗服务现状研究[J].潍坊工程职业学院学报,2015(4)：67—69.

[12]　国家卫生和计划生育委员会.中国卫生和计划生育统计年鉴2016[M].北京：中国协和医科大学出版社,2016：336.

[13]　郝君富,李心愉.德国长期护理保险：制度设计、经济影响与启示[J].人口学刊,2014(2)：104—112.

[14]　郝丽燕,杨士林.德国社会护理保险制度的困境与未来发展方向[J].德国研究,2015(2)：100—113.

[15]　何香,朱海萍,刘华玲,等.失能老年人照顾者护理负担的研究[J].中国护理管理,2014(5)：503—505.

[16]　黄婷婷. 我国人口老龄化对卫生总费用增长的影响[D]. 厦门：厦门大学, 2012.

[17]　蒋艳,赵丽颖,满晓玮,等.2002—2014年北京市卫生总费用医疗机构费用及药品费用流向分析[J].中国卫生经济,2016,35(5)：45—47.

[18]　焦翔,侯佳乐,田卓平.上海市老年护理供需测算与长期护理制度建设研究[J].中国医院管理,2014,34(7)：24—29.

[19]　解垩.与收入相关的健康及医疗服务利用不平等研究[J].经济研究,2009(2)：92—105.

[20]　李乐乐,张知新,王辰. 德国医疗保险制度对我国统筹发展的借鉴与思考[J]. 中国医院管理,2016,36(11)：94—96.

[21]　李矛.我国商业健康保险市场发展现状的研究报告——以四大专业健康保险公司为例[D].北京：对外经济贸易大学,2014.

[22]　李滔,张帆.德国医疗卫生体制改革现状与启示[J].中国卫生经济,2015(4)：92—96.

[23]　刘纯,尚尔宁,邵志高.英国医院临床药学服务模式初探[J].药学服务与研究,2015,15(5)：347—350.

[24]　刘继同.“一个制度、多种标准”与全民性基本医疗保险制度框架[J].人文杂志,2006(3)：7—13.

[25]　刘权,邓勇.德国医疗卫生体制的新变与启示[J].中国医院院长,2016(15)：66—71.

[26]　刘疏影,陈彪.帕金森病流行现状[J].中国现代神经疾病杂志,2016(2)：

98—101.

[27]　刘源,赵晶晶.德国的医疗保险和护理保险[J].保险研究,2008(3):
　　　89—91.

[28]　吕学静.日本医疗点数付费方式及借鉴[J].中国医疗保险,2010(6):
　　　58—59.

[29]　罗仁夏.10万元以上医疗保险住院病例医疗费用肥西[J].中国卫生资
　　　源,2005(6):41—42.

[30]　马爱霞,许扬扬.我国老年人医疗卫生支出影响因素研究[J].中国卫生
　　　政策研究,2015,8(7):68—73.

[31]　马里恩·卡斯佩斯—梅尔克.德国的卫生体制——特点、问题与解决方
　　　案[J].社会保障研究,2006(2):106—112.

[32]　牟蘋.综合医院药品费用分析与政策研究[D].北京:北京中医药大
　　　学,2010.

[33]　 彭佳平.上海市老年护理供需现状及对策研究[D].上海:复旦大
　　　学,2011.

[34]　饶克勤,钱军程,陈红敬,等.我国人口老龄化对卫生系统的挑战及其应
　　　对策略[J].中华健康管理学杂志,2012,6(1):6—8.

[35]　上海市统计局.2016上海统计年鉴[M].北京:中国统计出版社,2016.

[36]　施巍巍,刘一姣.德国长期照护保险制度研究及其启示[J].商业研究,
　　　2011(3):98—105.

[37]　史薇.荷兰老龄政策的经验与启示[J].老龄科学研究,2014,2(4):
　　　70—79.

[38]　隋学礼.德国医保筹资制度的改革路径分析——基于人口老龄化和家
　　　庭政策视角[J].北京航空航天大学学报(社会科学版),2016(2):
　　　13—19.

[39]　王丙毅,尹音频.德国医疗管制模式的特点、改革取向及借鉴意义[J].
　　　理论学刊,2008(7):58—61.

[40]　王超群.老龄化是卫生费用增长的决定性因素吗?[J].人口与经济,
　　　2014(3):23—30.

[41]　王鸿春,马仲良,鹿春江.民生策论:关于转变医疗模式政策的研究[J].
　　　资治文摘(管理版),2009(1):62—63.

[42]　王敏,李彦,孙晓阳.长期护理保险筹资机制研究——以德国和日本经

验为例[J].医学与法学,2017,9(1)：49—54.

[43] 王荣欣,秦俭,汤哲.我国老年人医疗服务现状及医疗服务需求[J].中国老年学杂志,2011(3)：534—536.

[44] 王翌秋,王舒娟.居民医疗服务需求及其影响因素微观实证分析的研究进展[J].中国卫生政策研究,2010(8)：55—62.

[45] 魏鹏.德国分级医疗体系管窥[J].中国医疗保险,2011(9)：70.

[46] 吴怀阳,王财元,郭红霞.影响住院费用若干因素分析[J].中国医院统计,2004,11(2)：138—139.

[47] 吴君槐.荷兰医保独树一帜[J].中国卫生,2015(4)：110—111.

[48] 谢春艳,金春林,王贤吉.英国整合型保健发展经验及启示[J].中国卫生资源,2015,18(1)：71—74.

[49] 许燕君,杨颖华,杨光,等.上海市老年护理床位配置现状及问题[J].中国卫生资源,2014(3)：157—159.

[50] 杨光,杨颖华,许燕君,等.上海市老年护理体系存在的突出问题探索[J].中国卫生资源,2014(3)：160—162.

[51] 杨颖华.上海市老年护理服务现状及对策研究[D].上海：复旦大学,2011.

[52] 于建明.德国的长期护理服务体系及启示[J].中国民政,2017(3)：57—58.

[53] 余红星,冯友梅,付旻,等.医疗机构分工协作的国际经验及启示——基于英国、德国、新加坡和美国的分析[J].中国卫生政策研究,2014(6)：10—15.

[54] 余央央.老龄化对中国医疗费用的影响——城乡差异的视角[J].世界经济文汇.2011(5)：64—78.

[55] 袁彩霞.我国老年长期护理保险制度实施路径研究[D].南京：南京师范大学,2014.

[56] 袁文蔚.我国老年护理消费需求与购买力分析[D].北京：清华大学,2013.

[57] 翟绍果.韩国国民健康保险费用偿付制度概览[J].中国医疗保险,2012(7)：70—72.

[58] 张涵,吴炳义,董惠玲.不同类型养老机构老年人医疗服务现状及需求调查[J].中国全科医学,2015(15)：1786—1790.

[59] 张强,高向东.老年人口长期护理需求及影响因素分析——基于上海调查数据的实证分析[J].西北人口,2016(2):87—90.

[60] 赵莹,郭林.荷德法三国医疗保障筹资改革[J].中国社会保障,2014(10):36—37.

[61] 周国伟.中国老年人自评自理能力:差异与发展[J].南方人口,2008(1):51—58.

[62] 周建再,代宝珍.德国慢性病管理现状[J].中国社会保障,2016(12):75—77.

[63] 周耀虹.社区社会组织参与社会服务的途径与价值探析[R].社会管理法治化理论与实践研讨会,2012.

英文文献

[1] Alemayehu B, Warner K E.The lifetime distribution of health care costs[J].Health Serv Res, 2004, 39: 627—642.

[2] Allen K, Bednarik R, Campbell L, et al. Governance and finance of long-term care across Europe, Overview Paper [R]. United Kingdom/Vienna: University of Birmingham/European Centre for Social Welfare Policy and Research: Birmingham, 2011.

[3] Barnato A E, McClellan M B, Garber C, et al. Trends in inpatient treatment intensity among medicare beneficiaries at the end of life [J]. Health Services Research, 2004, 39(2): 363—376.

[4] Becker G S. Human Capital [M]. New York: Columbia University Press (for Nat. Bur. Econ. Res.), 1964.

[5] Bettio F, Verashchagina A. Long-term care for the elderly. Provisions and providers in 33 European countries. Rome: Fondazione G, Brodolini, 2010.

[6] Bjørner T B, Arnberg S. Terminal costs, improved life expectancy and future public health expenditure[J]. International Journal of Health Care Finance and Economics, 2012, 12(2): 129—143.

[7] Blakely T, Atkinson J, Kvizhinadze G, et al. Health system costs by sex, age and proximity to death, and implications for estimation of future expenditure[J]. New Zealand Medical Journal, 2014, 127(1393): 12—25.

［8］ Brockmann H. Why is less money spent on health care for the elderly than for the rest of the population? Health care rationing in German hospitals［J］. Social Science and Medicine, 2002, 55(4): 593—608.

［9］ Brooks-Wilson A R. Genetics of healthy aging and longevity［J］. Human Genetics, 2013, 132(12): 1323—1338.

［10］ Buchner F, Wasem J. "Steeping" health expenditure profiles［J］. Geneva Papers on Risk & Insurance Issues & Practice, 2006, 31(4): 581—589.

［11］ Busse R, Blümel M. Germany: Health system review ［J］. Health Systems in Transition, 2014, 16(2): 1—296.

［12］ Commission on Social Determinants of Health. Closing the gap in a generation: health equity through action on social determinants of health. Final report of the Commission on Social Determinants of Health. Geneva: World Health Organization, 2008.

［13］ Crilly J, Chaboyer W, Wallis M. A structure and process evaluation of an Australian hospital admission avoidance programme for agedcare facility residents. Journal of Advanced Nursing, 2012, 68(2): 322—334.

［14］ Culter D M, Meara E. The medical costs of the young and old: A forty-year perspective［M］. Chicago: University of Chicago Press. 1998: 215—246.

［15］ de Vries M, Kossen J. How does the healthcare market operate? This is how Dutch healthcare works ［M］. Netherlands: De Argumentenfabriek, 2015.

［16］ Department of Health. End of Life Care Strategy: Promoting high quality care for adults at the end of their life［R］. 2008.

［17］ Dormonta B, Grignon M, Huber H. Health expenditure growth: Reassessing the threat of ageing ［J］. Health Econ. Health Economics, 2006, 15(9): 947—963.

［18］ Farrar S, Sussex J, Yi D, et al. National evaluation payment by results: Report to the department of Health［R］. UK: 2007: 6—8.

［19］ Felder S, Meier M, Schmitt H. Health care expenditure in the last months of life［J］. Journal of Health Economics, 2000, 19(5): 679—695.

［20］ Fuchs V R. Some economic aspects of mortality in the United States.

mimeographed[M]. New York: Nat. Bur. Econ. Res., 1965.

[21] Gozalo P, Plotzke M, Mor V. Changes in medicare costs with the growthof hospice care in nursing homes [J]. New England Journal of Medicine,2015, 372(19): 1823—1831.

[22] Grossman M. On the concept of health capital and the demand for health[J]. Journal of Political Economy, 1972, 80(2): 223—255.

[23] Hartman M, Catlin A, Lassman D, et al. U.S. Health spending by age, selected years through 2004[J]. Health Affairs, 2008, 27(1): w1—w12.

[24] Hartman M, Catlin A, Lassman D, et al.U.S.health spending by age, selected years through 2004[J].Health Affairs, 2008, 27(1).

[25] Hashimoto H, Ikegami N, Shibuya K, et al. Cost containment and quality of care in Japan: is there a trade-off? [J]. Lancet, 2011, 378 (9797): 1174—1182.

[26] Healthcare. The medical system. https: //www. justlanded. com / english/Netherlands/Netherlands-Guide/Health/Healthcare. (2017-6-29).

[27] Kerr C W, Donohue K A, Tangeman J C, et al. Cost savings and enhanced hospice enrollment with a home-based palliative care program implemented as a hospice-private payer partnership[J]. Journal of palliative medicine, 2014, 17(12): 1328—1335.

[28] Lassman D, Hartman M, Washington B, et al.US health spending trends by age and gender: Selected years 2002—10[J].Health Aff (Millwood), 2014,33(5): 815—822.

[29] Lubitz J D, Rily G F. Trends in Medicare payments in the last year of life[J]. New England Journal of Medicine, 1993, 328(15): 1092—1097.

[30] May P, Garrido M M, Cassel J B, et al. Prospective cohort study of hospital palliative care teams for inpatients with advanced cancer: Earlier consultation is associated with larger cost-saving effect[J]. Journal of Clinical Oncology, 2015, 33(25): 2745—2752.

[31] McCarthy I M, Robinson C, Huq S, et al. Cost savings from palliative care teams and guidance for a financially viable palliative care program[J]. Health services research, 2015, 50(1): 217—236.

[32] McGrail K, Bo Green, Barer M L, et al. Age, costs of acute and

long-term care and proximity to death: evidence for 1987—1988 and 1994—1995 in British Columbia[J]. Age and Ageing, 2000,29(3): 249—253.

[33] Ministry of Public Health, Welfare and Sport. Healthcare in the Netherlands, https: //www. government. nl /documents /leaflets / 2016 /02 /09 /healthcare-in-the-netherlands. (2018-1-8).

[34] Mot E, et al. The long-term care system for the elderly in the Netherlands. Netherlands: Enepri research report NO. 90 [R].2010, ISBN 978 9461380326.

[35] Mushkin S J. Health as an Investment. Journal of Political Economy, 1962(70): 129.

[36] O'Neill C, Groom L, Avery A J, et al. Age and proximity to death as predictors of GP care costs: results from a study of nursing home patients[J].Health Econmics,2000, 9(8): 733—738.

[37] Perls T T. Acute care costs of the oldest old[J]. Hospital Practice, 1997, 32(7): 123—137.

[38] Polder J J, Barendregt J J, Van O H. Health care costs in the last year of life-the Dutch experience[J]. Social Science & Medicine, 2006, 63(7): 1720—1731.

[39] Prince M J, Wu F, Guo Y, et al. The burden of disease in older people and implications for health policy and practice.Lancet[J]. 2015,385(9967): 549—562.

[40] Reinhardt U E.Does the aging of the population really drive the demand for health care? [J]. Health Affairs (Millwood), 2003, 22: 27—39.

[41] Riley G, Lubitz J, Prihoda R, et al. The use and costs of Medicare services by cause of death[J]. Inquiry, 1987, 24(3): 233—244.

[42] Rolden H J A, Rohling J H T, van Bodegom D, et al. Seasonal variation in Mortality, Medical care expenditure and institutionalization in older people: Evidence from a Dutch cohort of older health insurance clients [J]. PLOS One, 2015, 10(11): 1—14.

[43] Rolden H. The Dutch health care system [EB/OL]. Lyden Academy.

[44] Schultz T W. Investment in human capital[J]. American Economic Review, 1961, 51(1): 1—17.

[45] Schut E, Sorbe S Høj J. Health care reform and long-term care in the

Netherlands [R]. OECD Economics Department Working Papers, 2013, No. 1010.

[46] Serup-Hansen N, Wickstrom J, Kristiansen I S. Future health care costs—Do health care costs during the last year of life matter? [J]. Health Policy, 2002, 62(2): 161—172.

[47] Seshamani M, Bird C E, Schuster C R. Ageing and health-care expenditure: The red herring argument revisited [J]. Health Economics, 2004, 13(4): 303—314.

[48] Seshamani M, Gray A. Ageing and health-care expenditure: The red herring argument revisited[J]. Health Economics, 2004, 13(4): 303.

[49] Seshamani M, Gray A. Time to death and health expenditure: An improved model for the impact of demographic change on health care costs[J]. Age and ageing. 2004, 33(6): 556—561.

[50] Shugarman L R, Bird C E, Schuster C R, et al. Age and gender differences in medicare expenditures and service utilization at the end of life for lung cancer decedents.[J]. Womens Health Issues, 2008, 18(3): 199.

[51] Shugarman L R, Campbell D E, Bird C E, et al. Differences in Medicare expenditures during the last 3 years of life.[J]. Journal of General Internal Medicine, 2004, 19(2): 127—135.

[52] Spillman B C, Lubitz J. The effect of longevity on spending for acute and long-term care[J]. New England Journal of Medicine, 2000, 342 (19): 1409—1415.

[53] Temkingreener H, Meiners M R, Petty E A, et al. The use and cost of health services prior to death: A comparison of the Medicare-only and the Medicare-Medicaid elderly populations. [J]. Milbank Quarterly, 1992, 70(4): 679—701.

[54] Waldo D R, Lazenby H C.Demographic characteristics and health care use and expenditures by the aged in the United States: 1977—1984[J].Health Care Financing Review, 1984, 6(1): 1—29.

[55] Werblow A, Felder S, Zweifel P, et al. Population ageing and health care expenditure: A school of 'red herrings'? [J]. Health Economics, 2007, 16(10): 1109—1126.

[56] Wong A, van Baal P H, Boshuizen H C, et al. Exploring the influence of proximity to death on disease-specific hospital

expenditures：A carpaccio of red herrings［J］. Health Economics，2011，20(4)：379—400.

［57］ Yip W C，Hsiao W C，Chen W，et al. Early appraisal of China's huge and complex health-care reforms ［J］. Lancet，2012，379（9818）：833—842.

［58］ Zweifel P，Felder S，Meiers M. Ageing of population and health care expenditure：A red herring? ［J］. Health Economics，1999，8（6）：485—496.